The

PAIN
GAP

The

PAIN
GAP

HOW SEXISM
and RACISM
in HEALTHCARE
KILL WOMEN

ANUSHAY HOSSAIN

TILLER PRESS

NEW YORK   LONDON   TORONTO   SYDNEY   NEW DELHI

TILLER PRESS

An Imprint of Simon & Schuster, Inc.
1230 Avenue of the Americas
New York, NY 10020

First Tiller Press hardcover edition October 2021

TILLER PRESS and colophon are registered
trademarks of Simon & Schuster, Inc.

For information about special discounts for bulk purchases,
please contact Simon & Schuster Special Sales at 1-866-506-1949
or business@simonandschuster.com.

The Simon & Schuster Speakers Bureau can bring authors to your live event. For more
information or to book an event, contact the Simon & Schuster Speakers Bureau at
1-866-248-3049 or visit our website at www.simonspeakers.com.

Interior design by Laura Levatino

Manufactured in the United States of America

1   3   5   7   9   10   8   6   4   2

Library of Congress Cataloging-in-Publication Data has been applied for.

ISBN 978-1-9821-7777-5
ISBN 978-1-9821-7778-2 (ebook)

This book is dedicated to my grandfather,
Tofazzal Hossain Manik Miah, and to the love of my life,
Shy Pahlevani, and our daughters, Ava and Layla.

Contents

Foreword

Jessica Valenti

Ten years ago, I walked into my ob-gyn's office for what I thought would be a normal exam. I was a little under twenty-eight weeks pregnant and due to get my glucose exam. Sure, I had noticed that my feet and face were quite swollen—but it was August in New York! Who wouldn't be a bit puffy? I felt okay and thought I was fine.

But when the nurse took my blood pressure, a look of concern came over her face. She called in my doctor, who took it again. They turned the lights off in the room, told me to lie down and relax—to try to calm down—and that they would take my blood pressure one last time after five minutes.

It was after that third blood pressure reading that it became clear I was far from the healthy, glowing pregnant woman I imagined myself to be. My doctor told me I needed to leave her office and check myself into the hospital across the street. "Don't stop anywhere," she said. "Go right now."

Even after I was admitted a mere ten minutes later, my husband and I thought it all must be a fluke—a mistake of some kind. After all, I didn't *feel* sick, and we had months to go before our daughter was meant to be due. So when the head of obstetrics told us that I wouldn't be leaving the hospital until I delivered my baby, we were dumbstruck. I asked if I would really be in the hospital for three whole months. His reply landed like a punch to the gut: "We'll be happy if you make it a week."

I was diagnosed with severe preeclampsia, a dangerous condition that causes high blood pressure in pregnant women—if left untreated, it can lead to seizures and death. Soon, we were surrounded by different doctors and specialists, each trying to get more information while letting us know what to expect.

One older male doctor suggested that I might be sick because of a previous abortion, that ending a pregnancy could be a cause of preeclampsia—something I found out later was absolutely untrue. Another man, who I had never been introduced to, came into my room at one point and stuck his fingers inside of me to see if my cervix was dilated. I never found out if he was a doctor, nurse, or why he needed to examine me at that moment.

I understood that things needed to move fast and that my health and pregnancy were in danger—but my personhood soon became secondary to the flurry of people and decisions that were being made around me.

Within two days of being admitted to the hospital, I developed a much more serious pregnancy complication—HELLP syndrome. My liver was in danger of failing, and we had to deliver my daughter immediately in order for me to live. I was rushed into an emergency C-section, and Layla was born weighing just two pounds, two ounces.

The next twenty-four hours were as close to hell as I could imagine. We waited hours to find out if my daughter was going to be okay, and even once we knew she was stable I was too sick to visit her. The medication I was on had me so confused that I kept asking my husband what our daughter's name was; I could hardly move because of the pain; and I was swollen with almost twenty pounds of water weight. (The swelling was so bad, in fact, that when a nurse tried to take blood her finger left an indent in my arm more than an inch deep.)

I thought I was going to die, and almost twenty-four hours after delivering, when I saw how little Layla was, I thought she was going to die, too.

In the end, miraculously, we were both all right. I slowly recovered, and so did Layla—who had to spend eight weeks in the neonatal intensive care unit. It would be three years before her lungs and immune system recovered, and even longer before I was reasonably over the trauma that came along with watching your child almost die with you close behind. If I'm being honest, I don't know that I ever truly "got over" it.

This experience, this series of moments that shifted my life forever, is part of the reason I'm so passionate about *The Pain Gap* and the issues it examines.

It's incredibly difficult to explain to people who haven't been sick before—really sick—how vulnerable you feel. How powerless you are. And how, in those minutes or days or weeks in a hospital or doctor's office, you are at the mercy of the people around you. And while those experts and professionals are generally smart and kind, they are also human—and prone to the same foibles and biases as the rest of us.

Being a woman in America is already fraught; being a sick woman in America is doubly difficult. You aren't believed, or you're condescended to. Your pain is treated as hysteria, your physical symptoms as signs of mental duress rather than authentic illness. For women who aren't white, or straight, or upper middle class, the judgment is that much harsher and the consequences that much more serious.

My experience in the hospital was traumatizing—but I was still believed and taken care of. My illness was caught early enough to save my life and my daughter's. My outcome would have been a lot different if I wasn't a white, well-off woman with insurance who was admitted to a prestigious and well-funded hospital.

We're in the middle of a maternal health crisis for Black women: mothers with the very same disease I had ten years ago are dying and their babies along with them. Their pain is being dismissed and their symptoms ignored. They are being called difficult and aggressive. They are dying of diseases that we know how to stop.

I cannot imagine, in the middle of the most painful and terrifying experience of your life, having to deal with the extra fear and burden of having to convince people that you are, in fact, sick. That you need help.

That's why *The Pain Gap* is so important—it shines a light on the disparity of care in this country. And it shows women how they can best advocate for themselves and their loved ones.

We're living in a moment—post–Me Too and post-Trump—when the issues impacting women are in danger of being brushed aside. But the urgency is far from over. And I can't think of a more vital and consequential place to start interrogating inequality than the spaces—doctor's offices, hospitals, clinics—where our literal lives are in other people's hands.

The

PAIN
GAP

As a general rule, all women are hysterical. And every woman carries with her the seeds of hysteria.[1]

—Dr. Auguste Fabre, physician, 1883

We are volcanoes. When we women offer our experience as our truth, as human truth, all the maps change. There are new mountains. That's what I want—to hear you erupting. You young Mount St. Helenses who don't know the power in you—I want to hear you.[2]

—Ursula K. Le Guin, author, 1986

Introduction

When I became pregnant in the United States, I was so relieved. Having grown up in Bangladesh in the 1980s, where the concept of women's health hardly existed and dying in childbirth was a common occurrence, I knew how lucky I was to be able to access the best healthcare in the world. I trusted the doctors and nurses implicitly with my health and my baby's life.

I could not have been more mistaken.

Things went awry from the minute I got to the hospital, and after thirty hours of labor, three of which I spent pushing, my epidural slipped. My pain was so severe that I ran a fever of 104 degrees, and as I shook and trembled uncontrollably, the doctors finally performed an emergency C-section.

While all the commotion, fear, and pain took me by surprise, I kept telling myself over and over, "I am in America. I will be fine. I know I am not going to die in childbirth in Washington, DC!"

But it wasn't until later that I realized how naive I had been. That day, I came dangerously close to losing both my life and my baby's. The experience was traumatic and left me with severe hyperthyroidism. I developed a condition called Graves' disease, where my thyroid levels were through the roof and my left eye began to protrude. The struggle women go through every day to give birth safely suddenly became a tangible reality for me.

Despite my years as a feminist policy analyst on Capitol Hill, working on global health legislation, it took almost dying on the delivery room table for me to see that pregnancy-related deaths are not merely casualties of the so-called developing world.

But what plagues me most is why I stayed so uncharacteristically quiet through it all. Why, when I insisted the painkillers weren't working and everyone was ignoring me, did I not once raise my voice? Why, after I was in surgery, was I so polite to the doctor who demanded I "prove" my pain by walking to the operating table on my own? Where was my voice—the "hysteria" I had used selectively and to my advantage in the past? Having spent my entire career as a women's rights advocate, why didn't I stand up for myself?

"Hysteria"—it's hard to think of a word in the English language with roots more sexist than this ancient Greek word for "uterus." Not surprisingly, the first person to describe female hysteria was a man. The Greek physician Hippocrates, often called the Father of Medicine, believed that the uterus was a "free-floating, wandering animal" that moved through the female body, causing a host of problems when it bumped into other organs.

Medically, the term "hysteria" is defined gender-neutrally, as a "general state of extreme fear and panic." But the word remains inextricably linked to women. (Just try to think of the last time you heard a man described as "hysterical.")

Feminist author Mona Eltahawy compares "hysteria" to other words which shame the victim instead of the abuser.

"Words like 'riot' and 'chaos' are like 'hysterical' when the latter is used to describe a woman's justified frustration and rage against sexism and misogyny," Eltahawy said. "Those words shift judgement away from the oppressor to the oppressed."[3]

Even though the pseudoscience behind this made-up condition has been largely debunked, the concept of hysteria characterizes women's medical diagnoses to this day. Doctors still don't always believe women when they describe their pain, or they dismiss women's symptoms as being psychosomatic. All in all, healthcare in America carries some serious sexist baggage.

And it has serious consequences. The list of examples of how misogyny in medical practice profoundly impacts women's health is endless. Heart disease is the leading killer of American women, but because it's still thought of as a "male disease," women are less likely to be diagnosed accurately when they have a heart attack.[4] Women make up the majority of those suffering from chronic-pain disorders, but doctors are more likely to refer them to a therapist than prescribe adequate pain medication. America's maternal mortality numbers are the highest in the industrialized world—partly because doctors simply don't believe women when they say they're in pain.

And if you're a woman of color, things are even worse. Heart disease and stroke are the leading causes of death for all American women, but the majority of people dying are Black women, with more than 60 percent living with some form of heart complication.[5]

The image of motherhood in America is often that of a white woman, but it's women of color who are two to three times more likely to die from pregnancy-related causes.[6] For years, everything from education level to socioeconomic background were blamed for these massive racial disparities, but now experts are finally pointing to racism—not race—as the biggest driving factor.

Giving birth in the richest country on earth, I never imagined I could die in labor. But I almost did. The experience put me on a journey to explore, understand, and share how women—especially women of color—are dismissed to death by systemic sexism in American healthcare.

This book is about the journey of learning to own my hysteria and rebrand it for the twenty-first century. It is the story of growing up in Bangladesh, surrounded by staggering maternal mortality rates, before lobbying for global health legislation on Capitol Hill and nearly becoming a maternal mortality statistic myself—all the while blissfully unaware of how dangerous it can be just to go to the hospital as a woman in America.

This book encourages women to embrace the power of their "hysteria" and redefine it as a positive response—a way to summon their voices instead of staying silent. A way to demand a response, a reaction.

Women should stop letting the legacy of hysteria silence and shame us. Instead, we should repurpose its deeply sexist history as a way to advocate for our own health. After centuries of having our symptoms dismissed and being told we're crazy, have we not earned the right to speak out—in effect, to get "hysterical"?

When it comes to our health and rights, the truth is women aren't being hysterical *enough*. Throughout history, we have been too quiet. We are still staying silent and polite—and it's literally killing us.

Perhaps a little fury and confrontation is just what the doctor ordered. And that's exactly what this book is all about.

Following in the footsteps of feminist manifestos such as *The Feminine Mystique* and *Rage Becomes Her*, *The Pain Gap* is an eye-opening call to arms that encourages women to flip our hysteria complex on its head and use it to bring about the women's health revolution we need.

This book presents a compelling argument for urgent change while arming women—especially women of color—with a guide to their bodies and complaints, so that they have the support, information, and confidence to be their own best health advocates.

Meticulously researched and grounded in in-depth reportage of real women's tales of healthcare trauma and medical misogyny, *The Pain Gap* illustrates how America got to this women's health crisis point—and what women can do about it.

1

The First Feminist
I Ever Knew

When I was a little girl growing up in Bangladesh in the 1980s, my mother was very involved with the women's rights movement, and she used to take me with her everywhere. As the youngest of her four daughters, I was my mom's constant companion.

When Ammu (Bengali for "mom") started the country's first women's rights magazine, I did my homework sitting at her desk in the back office. When she opened a school for underprivileged Bangladeshi girls, I held her hand at the ribbon-cutting ceremony. Ammu was the first feminist I ever knew, and although I didn't realize it at the time, she was nurturing my feminist soul along with her own.

Perhaps because I had gotten so used to accompanying my mom to her activist events, it wasn't until my sophomore year of high school that it clicked for me just how radical it was to fight for women's rights in a country like Bangladesh.

In 1996, when I was sixteen years old, my father won two seats[1] in the Bangladeshi Parliament and was also appointed by the prime minister as a cabinet minister. Abbu (Bengali for "father") was approaching the zenith of his political career, where he would remain for the next two decades.

In a move both strategic and bold, he nominated my mother for one of his seats, giving her some serious clout of her own, and turning them into a political power couple. Ammu had to beat out two male rivals, but she won the district that year and became a member of Parliament (MP) in the Bangladeshi government.

At the time, in the capital of Dhaka, there was a growing debate over the rights of sex workers. Prostitution in Bangladesh is legal if the brothels are licensed, but most aren't. In the mid-1990s, brothels in the city were routinely raided by the local police, who would set fire to the slums where they operated.

The majority of sex workers were young women and underage girls who had been trafficked into the city and sold into prostitution. With the brothels ablaze, they had nowhere to go.

When they began pouring onto the main roads and into city centers, they were horrifically beaten and publicly assaulted by the very same law enforcement officers who had raided the brothels in the first place. Police mutilated many of the women's faces with knives, gouging their flesh to mark, humiliate, and scar them permanently.

But advocating for sex workers in a Muslim country was not a cause that most women's rights groups wanted to get involved in. So, when it was time for Ammu to give her first speech in Parliament after being sworn in as the representative of the Bangladeshi district of Pirojpur in Barisal, she took the opportunity to spotlight this issue, framing it as a crisis of violence against Bangladeshi women.

As my mom approached the microphone, I watched from a small wooden balcony in a tucked-away private room overlooking the Commons Chamber of Parliament. On the floor of the Bangladeshi government, dominated by manspreading lawmakers, my mom stood up at the podium and beamed under the bright lights. Her head loosely covered with the dupata of her light pink sari, Ammu proposed amending the law in order to protect the rights of sex workers.

Afterward, my mom had a group of the workers over to celebrate at our family home in Dhanmondi, just a stone's throw from the Houses of Parliament. Ammu was always good about opening up our home to all kinds of people, especially those not as privileged as we were, perhaps because she herself had grown up with so little.

That day, our formal living room was packed with women in their neon-colored saris, matching bright makeup, and shimmering glass bangles. In the center of it all, playing hostess and making sure everyone's teacups and plates were full, was Ammu. I wandered about the festive and colorful chaos, trying to go unnoticed, when a young woman named Shamoli, clad in a bright yellow sari and matching floral blouse, took me aside.

"Your mother is the first person to treat us like human beings, Apu," she said, referring to me as "sister" in Bengali. I leaned in to hug her when Shamoli took my hand and placed it over a scar that ran right from the corner of her eye to her mouth.

In many ways, my mom's work was making us all, including me, aware of our rights (or lack thereof) as Bangladeshi women. Watching Ammu take on the plight of sex workers, run an election campaign, and continue the fight all the way to the government not only showed me what my mom was made of but how dangerous it was to be a woman in an über-patriarchal society like ours.

It made me see how far women had to go to protect our fragile rights, and how difficult those rights were to access in the first place. It also revealed how openly women were allowed to be treated as less than, even subhuman, in our country. But perhaps most strikingly, the experience made me see that in a country where women were overwhelmingly powerless, Ammu was not. Unfortunately, it would not take long to discover the limits of her power.

In South Asian culture, having domestic servants was not a luxury reserved for the wealthy. Bangladesh was no exception. In very lucky cases, the family you work for provides you with medical care. My mom made sure our staff was taken care of—cleaners, cooks, nannies, and general staff. But the needs of my beloved childhood nanny, Wasifa, were anything but ordinary.

Wasifa worked for our family for about fourteen years. Although her main task was to take care of my older sister, Maneeza, and me, she was "my" nanny from the time I was three years old until I turned seventeen. The two of us were so close that my siblings still joke that as a kid I probably thought Wasifa was my mother. And, in so many ways, she was.

When I had bad dreams, I crawled out of my bed to the floor, where, most nights, Wasifa would be sleeping. If I needed a glass of water in the middle of the night, I would go to Wasifa. When I was six years old, there was a short period when I couldn't walk. Wasifa carried me on her hip like a baby until I regained mobility.

Wasifa made all my meals growing up. I remember how she would roll her special chicken curry and basmati rice into perfect little balls just for me. I cannot count how many late afternoons we spent on the rooftop, me sitting with my head against Wasifa's knees, listening to her tell stories while she braided my hair, the loud Dhaka traffic blaring as a burning orange sun set into the monsoon sky.

When Wasifa got married, things quickly went south. From the beginning of their union, her husband put a lot of pressure on her to not only get pregnant but also to produce a boy. Wasifa was diabetic, which complicated her efforts. As soon as she got pregnant for the first time, Wasifa miscarried—the beginning of a series of painful miscarriages that made her weaker and weaker, right before our eyes.

I often came home from school to find Wasifa sleeping or weeping quietly in some corner of the house. One day, I found her hunched over in the kitchen, bleeding through her sari, whimpering in pain. I screamed for my mom, and we rushed her to the nearest hospital.

"Your pregnancies will be the death of you," Dr. Iqbal Wahab warned Wasifa as we sat with her in the hospital room. "You must stop trying for a baby."

Dr. Wahab explained that because of her diabetes, Wasifa's high blood-glucose levels made it more likely that she would miscarry, and that even if she managed to carry a pregnancy to term, the chances of a stillbirth, or worse, were high. Ironically, not long after those dire warnings, Wasifa got pregnant again. But this time, to everyone's surprise, she carried to term, and finally gave birth to the baby boy she wanted so badly.

I was still at school when I got the news that Wasifa had delivered. I could hardly wait to go to the hospital to meet this baby! I felt as if I had gotten a little brother. Wasifa was finally a mother! I still remember all the plans I was making of how I was going to dress the baby, feed him, and make him my little doll.

Despite a relatively normal delivery, Wasifa had heavy postpartum bleeding and hemorrhaged so much that her blood pressure dropped sharply—a lethal combination for any woman after birth. By the time school ended that day, Wasifa was dead. She had named her son Farooq.

Losing Wasifa was a turning point in my seventeen-year-old life. It changed who I was, and though I didn't realize it at the time, it transformed me into a women's rights activist. It humanized the issue of maternal health and rendered me incapable of ever viewing maternal mortality statistics as just numbers on a page.

Wasifa's death also made it impossible to ignore that for the vast majority of women in Bangladesh, access to healthcare was based on pure luck, and even then, it couldn't save you. The women who worked in our home got access to whatever medical care they could through my mom, but Ammu had access only because she herself was married to a rich and powerful man—my father.

It wasn't enough to save Wasifa, and it wasn't enough to save the hundreds of thousands of women dying in pregnancy-related deaths in a country where the concept of women's rights was still so controversial.

That said, Wasifa's death coincided with major changes about to be enacted on behalf of Bangladeshi women, especially on the family-planning and reproductive-rights front. Through most of the 1970s and '80s, Bangladesh had one of the world's highest maternal mortality rates, as well as exponential population growth. There were 120 million people in a country the size of the state of Wisconsin, mostly because women couldn't access family planning and contraceptives.[2]

But in 1994, the historic International Conference on Population and Development (ICPD) was held in Cairo, Egypt. The Cairo Conference, as it is commonly called, was the largest intergovernmental conference ever held on population and development. A total of eleven thousand participants came together to assemble the "Programme of Action," which underscored "the integral and mutually reinforcing linkages between population and development."[3] It was at this conference that the international community reached consensus on three key goals: the reduction of infant, child, and maternal mortality; the provision of universal access to education, particularly for girls; and the provision of universal access to a full range of reproductive health services, including family planning.[4]

This marked a turning point, when population policies stopped focusing on controlling and slowing population growth and explicitly addressed empowering women. The idea was that if women had access to education, contraceptives, and better-paying jobs, they would choose to have smaller families, thus lowering fertility rates.

"Not only did the ICPD consensus delegitimize top-down governmental efforts that ignored or violated women's human rights, it recognized that policies on development, in fact, could not succeed without ensuring such rights," a policy review paper from the Guttmacher Institute states. "Accordingly, the Programme of Action enumerated a set of principles related to nondiscrimination and free and informed decision making regarding the right to control one's own fertility."[5]

Between 1996 and 2004, Bangladesh made major progress in reducing the number of women dying in childbirth and pregnancy-related complications by bringing the maternal mortality numbers down from 514 per 100,000 live births between 1986 and 1990 to 322 per 100,000 live births between 1998 and 2000.[6]

Thanks in large part to now-iconic Bangladeshi nonprofits, such as the Grameen Bank and BRAC (Bangladesh Rural Advancement Committee), the country became a "development star," and a model for successful implementation of maternal health interventions. Over the next two decades, Bangladesh would go on to slash its maternal mortality rates by a whopping 40 percent.[7]

But none of this progress would bring Wasifa back. Soon after her death, her husband remarried and started a new life with his young bride. When we got the news from Wasifa's village, it pierced my heart. How could anyone move on from Wasifa so quickly?

Little did I know, my own life would soon start moving pretty fast, too. My older sister, Maneeza, was home for the summer from her first year at the University of Virginia. She insisted I attend a summer writing camp there.

Although my interest in journalism and writing was growing, leaving Bangladesh for such a camp did not interest me. I was still in mourning for Wasifa. But my sister was determined, and it didn't take much to convince my parents.

"You're going to be a senior in high school, and UVA is one of the best colleges in America."

I can still hear Maneeza doing her best to sell her younger sister on this grand plan.

"You have a real talent for writing, Anushay. Take it seriously."

She did not stop there. Maneeza pointed out how, while in Charlottesville, I could interview in person with the dean of admissions, Parke Muth, and if I liked UVA, I could apply for an early decision. My parents, of course, loved the idea of my getting a head start in the college-application process. Before I knew it, I was on a plane going halfway across the world.

It was a late-afternoon British Airways flight from Dhaka Zia International Airport flying direct to London and then to Washington. As the sun dipped below the horizon, I closed my eyes and thought about Wasifa. I thought about her huge Bette Davis eyes, how they took up half her face. She looked so much like the woman in Picasso's *Portrait of Françoise*—long, black, loose curls tousling past her waist.

Although I did not know it then, I was embarking on one of the most important journeys of my life—to the richest country in the world, where, almost fifteen years later, I would come close to dying in childbirth myself.

2

A Bangladeshi Girl
on Capitol Hill

When I first set foot on Capitol Hill, I had little idea of how the US government worked and even less about how policy was made. My knowledge of Bangladeshi politics, absorbed through my parents, did not prepare me for my first real job—as a lobbyist, right out of college in 2002. The US war in Afghanistan wasn't even a year old, and there was still an incredible amount of American political will to "liberate" the country from the Taliban, capture bin Laden, set up democracy, and deliver female empowerment to Afghan women and girls (draped in the US flag, of course). Hence my dream gig, as the project organizer for the Nobel Peace Prize–nominated Afghan Women and Girls Campaign, at the Feminist Majority Foundation (FMF). The United States may have invaded Afghanistan and ousted the Taliban from power in 2001 as retaliation for the September 11 attack on the World Trade Center, but it was the plight of Afghan women that the US government exploited to win the public relations and optics battle for the war with the American public.

It was very effective. Headlines everywhere shouted "Lift the Veil," or promised to give you a peek "Behind the Veil." All the rhetoric focused on freeing Afghan women from their evil Muslim male captors and blue-burqa prisons, and America—including me—just ate it up.

A *Time* magazine cover from 2001, which featured a carefully lit close-up of an Afghan woman's face, suggested how much better off Afghan women would be now that American boots were on the ground, from Kabul to Kandahar.[1]

"The fight against terrorism is also a fight for the rights and dignity of women," then First Lady Laura Bush said after the 2001 US invasion. Thanks to US intervention, she said, Afghan women were "no longer imprisoned in their homes."[2]

It is hard to imagine an American First Lady making such a statement today, but so soon after 9/11, the country's pain was palpable. People needed a reason for hope and optimism.

Understandably, the American public's trust of Muslims was also at an all-time low, and in many ways, Islamophobia had become part and parcel of US national security. This was when migrant detention facilities such as Guantánamo Bay were repurposed to hold detainees from the "war on terror" without due process.

This was also when my Arab American friends quietly dropped the "Abdel" from their names and became Ali Rahman instead of Ali Abdel-Rahman. All the Mohammeds I knew suddenly became "Mikes" or "Moes." I was regularly asked, when people learned my last name, if I were related to Iraq's Saddam Hussein.

While most Americans first learned about the Taliban after 9/11, for me it was 1996, as a teenager in Bangladesh. I vividly remember hearing on the news that armed men were forcing Afghan women into the all-enveloping blue burqas. I remember hearing that Afghan women doctors and engineers had suddenly been banned from the workplace. I remember the woman assassinated by Taliban bullets as she lay prostrate at the soccer stadium in Kabul, and how quickly the blood drenched her blue burqa.

I remember watching as the women of Afghanistan brutally vanished in front of the world's eyes—beaten to death by the butt end of a Talib rifle as bearded men waved shotguns and pistols at them. Men threw acid on the women for daring to show themselves outside their homes, and police officers whipped them for not standing behind their male guardians. I remember worrying that what was happening in Afghanistan could happen in Bangladesh, too.

And then came silence. The world unanimously—and quietly—decided to forget this nation in Central Asia, famously labeled by historians as the "graveyard of empires."[3] I heard nothing more about the Taliban until September 11, 2001.

Watching the Taliban return to the airwaves was like rediscovering an old terror I had not thought about since my schoolgirl days in Bangladesh. But now, degree in hand, I was a budding feminist determined to bring the fight to the real world.

That's what led me to the Feminist Majority Foundation's Afghan Women and Girls Campaign. Not only had the foundation been working in Afghanistan long before the US invasion, but they had just been nominated for the Nobel Peace Prize.

Securing Afghan women's rights was now the principal mission of my life. Maybe this was because I was unable to fight for them as a young girl. Maybe it was just believing with all my heart that if the Taliban were able to erase women from society and get away with it, no women anywhere would ever be truly safe. Maybe it was a bit of both.

The president and cofounder of the organization was American feminist icon Eleanor "Ellie" Smeal. The three-time National Organization of Women president played a key role in the movement to ratify the Equal Rights Amendment, and although I was unfamiliar with her work before I joined FMF, Ellie quickly became a very important person in my life and career.

It is not an overstatement to say that everything I learned about how Washington works, how policy works, activism, organizing, and feminism, I learned by Ellie's side. She became my mentor, and I loved her fiercely, even idolized her.

Her office was a sort of feminist Hollywood. It was not uncommon to bump into Gloria Steinem in the hallway, or Dolores Huerta at the holiday party. Working for Ellie Smeal and the FMF meant accompanying Angelina Jolie to the US State Department and briefing her on the latest anti–sex trafficking legislation. It meant seeing my boss sitting next to then senator Joe Biden during Barack Obama's Democratic National Convention speech in 2008, when he officially accepted the party's nomination. Biden and Ellie were and are very close, having worked together on the 1994 Violence Against Women Act (VAWA).

But it was the Afghan Women and Girls Campaign that put me on the Hill. That was the issue that introduced me to the world of policymaking and taught me how to lobby a bill—from its inception to authoring its language to convincing senators to support it to getting it to the floor for a vote.

Funding Afghan women–led organizations in Afghanistan; expanding the International Security Assistance Forces beyond just the capital, Kabul; and sponsoring dozens of Afghan refugees to attend college in America were all priorities for FMF's Afghan women campaign. And Ellie Smeal's strategy was always two-pronged—political action and educational advocacy—when it came to making sure US foreign policy protected and advocated for Afghan women's rights.

Once I was there, my lobbying portfolio quickly expanded. Before I knew it, I was working on other major legislation, such as the Convention on the Elimination of All Forms of Discrimination Against Women (CEDAW), and the International Violence Against Women Act (IVAWA). I went to briefings in the Russell building on the House side of the Hill, where, after hearing a panel on why America should ratify CEDAW, Senator Biden met with throngs of women's rights activists and advised us on how we could ensure our legislation got to the floor for a vote. I remember clearly his warning FMF staff that "family planning" had become a "poison pill" on Capitol Hill, synonymous with abortion, and to avoid the term when authoring legislation.

Biden was right. When I started representing the Feminist Majority in the Washington, DC, International Family Planning Coalition (IFPC), it didn't take long for me to see just how right.

The IFPC consisted of some of the top American reproductive health and rights organizations, who had serious political clout on Capitol Hill: the Guttmacher Institute, Population Action International, the United Nations Foundation, the Center for Reproductive Rights, and International Planned Parenthood Federation, among many others.

This broad coalition authored pro-family-planning language to be included in US funding legislation for international health programs and advocated for the United States to return to the goals laid out at the 1994 United Nations ICPD, which put women's empowerment at the heart of global population policy.

Why does the United States care about the reproductive health and rights of women around the world? It is estimated that more than 300,000 women and girls die from pregnancy- and childbirth-related complications, the majority of which occur in the so-called developing world. Approximately one-third of these deaths are preventable, especially with access to contraception. Experts estimate that worldwide, 214 million women have an unmet need for modern contraception.[4]

For more than fifty years, the US government has invested in international family-planning and reproductive health programs and is the funder of these efforts in the world. The United States is also one of the largest distributors and purchasers of contraceptives.[5]

According to a 2020 Congressional Research Service report, US foreign assistance, also called foreign aid, makes up the largest part of the international affairs budget. The roots of foreign aid go back to the European Recovery Program, also known as the Marshall Plan, that helped rebuild Europe after World War II.[6]

After the terrorist attacks of September 11, 2001, a large portion of US assistance focused on counterterrorism programs related to US military personnel in Iraq and Afghanistan. At the same time, global health assistance expanded significantly, with George W. Bush's PEPFAR (President's Emergency Plan for AIDS Relief) initiative to address the global HIV/AIDS epidemic. The size, composition, and purpose of foreign-assistance programs is decided by Congress, mainly through the appropriations process, and is reviewed annually.

Depending on which political party is in power, America's role in international family-planning efforts changes, especially on the issue of abortion. US funding for family planning/reproductive health is governed by a few legislative and policy restrictions, including a legal ban on the direct use of US funding overseas for abortion as a method of family planning, something that has been in effect since 1973. Working on the Hill gave me a front-row seat to how America exports its own abortion politics to the rest of the world.

In addition to lobbying with this coalition to increase US assistance to international family-planning programs, one of our major objectives was for the United States to repeal a policy called the Mexico City Policy, or the Global Gag Rule (GGR), an American policy that prohibits foreign nongovernmental organizations (NGOs) from "performing or actively promoting abortion as a method of family planning,"[7] the policy states, and using funds from *any* source (including non-US funds) as a condition of receiving US government global family-planning assistance.

Under the GGR, in order for an organization to remain eligible for US government funds, doctors, midwives, nurses, and civil society advocates cannot even mention the word "abortion"—much less provide abortion services—*even in countries where abortion is legal and a woman requests it.*

Organizations that choose not to meet these restrictions lose all US government funding, including that for essential supplies of contraceptives as well as technical assistance such as sonogram machines.[8]

"Organizations are presented with the choice to either give up talking about abortion or lose all of their US funding," Akila Radhakrishnan, president of the Global Justice Center, a New York City–based nonprofit, explained to *Vice*. "There are not a lot of organizations that have the ability to refuse US aid."[9]

It's important to note that the GGR is not just denying funding for abortion—it's a prohibition on *talking* about abortion as well. It is, quite literally, a gag order. Since 1973, the Helms Amendment has prohibited NGOs that receive federal funds from using those funds "to pay for the performance of abortions as a method of family planning."

Due to this amendment, the US government has maintained a de facto ban on funding abortion care with foreign-assistance dollars for more than forty years. But this wasn't restrictive enough for some GOP politicians who want to police language as well.

It's also important to point out that American NGOs are not required to make the same certifications, because the policy violates the constitutional right to free speech. Foreign NGOs, on the other hand, are considered fair game. It is criminal that in this day and age, US foreign assistance is blatantly weaponized to attack women's reproductive health and rights globally.

Though the official intention of the GGR is to reduce the number of abortions around the world, the Gag Rule has cruel consequences for the health and lives of poor women and their families.

Implementation of the Global Gag Rule resulted in people in Africa, Asia, and the Middle East losing US government–donated contraceptives, and many organizations and clinics have been forced to lay off staff or shut down altogether.[10] The result has been particularly devastating for women in rural areas, where there is often just one clinic providing an array of services, usually one receiving US funding.

The GGR was first formulated under the Reagan administration and has been rescinded and reinstated like clockwork by subsequent administrations along party lines. It was repealed by President Bill Clinton, reestablished by President George W. Bush, and rescinded again by President Barack Obama.

Under President Donald Trump, not only was the GGR reinstated in 2017, but *expanded* in 2019. The Trump administration's application of the policy extends to the vast majority of US bilateral global health assistance programs, including funding for HIV under PEPFAR, maternal and child health, malaria, nutrition, and other initiatives.

American women need to know and should be enraged about how US domestic abortion politics have spilled onto the international arena, creating barriers between women and their ability to access safe and legal abortions—*even if they are legal in their own countries*. There is perhaps no policy that demonstrates better than the GGR how disproportionately US domestic politics can affect everyone else.

But the Global Gag Rule is also not something we have to accept. American women should learn to get "hysterical" about it, because we can use our voices to change it—by organizing, lobbying, and joining the campaigns of hundreds of organizations that are already working on Capitol Hill to *permanently* repeal the GGR.

To this day, I am haunted by a very young pregnant girl I met in a clinic in Matlab, Bangladesh, during a nonwork-related trip. Moushumi was a domestic worker who had been raped by her employer, and her mother brought her to the clinic because she was complaining of intense stomach pains.

The girl and I sat in a thick, tangible silence in an unlit mud house as everyone around us made decisions on her behalf. She never looked up once. No one had the courage to tell this girl that terminating her pregnancy was an option, even though there was an abortion clinic literally across the street.

No one wanted to lose their American money or computers. They couldn't afford to. This girl had no choice but to have her baby, and she died soon after from pregnancy-related complications.

Stories like this don't just happen in Bangladesh. Research shows the consequences are both devastating and far-reaching. And in a perhaps predictable irony, it also suggests the GGR increases the rate of abortion.

A twenty-country study from Stanford University examining the Global Gag Rule in sub-Saharan Africa found that countries with "high exposure" to the policy experienced a relative decline in the use of modern contraceptives and an increase in the induced abortion rate. In Madagascar, health experts point out that the GGR is forcing women to choose between buying food or paying for contraceptives.[11]

Because so many providers are afraid to lose their funding if they have even a slight connection to an organization associated with abortion in any way, these policies create panic and end up making basic sexual and reproductive healthcare inaccessible in countries where women need fewer barriers to surmount, not more.

In recent years, Nepal and Kenya changed their abortion policy in an effort to reduce high maternal mortality rates because they recognized how unsafe abortions were needlessly killing women and girls.[12] Women in Nepal and Kenya experience high rates of sexual- and gender-based violence, but it is an American policy, like the GGR, that is preventing these countries from addressing this crisis.

We must end the Global Gag Rule. As was expected, one of the first actions President Biden took after coming to office was to immediately repeal the GGR, rescinding expansions that were made under the Trump administration. But that is not good enough. We need to *permanently* eliminate this policy and stop playing politics with women's health and reproductive rights—at home and abroad.

Although Médecins Sans Frontières (MSF) does not accept US government funding, the medical aid charity issued a statement after Biden repealed the GGR. The group spoke about the harm the policy had on limiting women's access to healthcare. In 2019, MSF treated more than 25,800 women and girls with abortion-related complications.[13]

"We've seen women who have used pens, broken glass, or sticks to try to induce an abortion," Dr. Manisha Kumar, head of MSF's task force on safe abortion care, said in a statement on the organization's website. "We've seen women who drank chlorine or poisons. . . . We can only guess how many women lost their lives over the last several years because access to this essential health care was cut off. And we know that policies such as the Global Gag Rule disproportionately affect black women and women of colour."[14]

As Americans, we have a responsibility to educate ourselves about how US foreign policy impacts women and girls globally because what happens here matters for women's rights around the world. When we vote in the United States, we are not only voting for ourselves. We are voting for women's rights globally. That's how powerful our politics and American policies are.

A 2020 study by the Guttmacher Institute, a leading research and policy organization committed to advancing sexual and reproductive health and rights in the United States, finds that 121 million women face an unintended pregnancy every year, meaning almost *half* of all pregnancies worldwide are unintended.[15] More than 60 percent of all unintended pregnancies end in abortion.

A 2016 analysis, also by the Guttmacher Institute, found that the US Agency for International Development budget for family planning gave twenty-seven million women and couples access to contraceptives, prevented more than two million unsafe abortions and six million unintended pregnancies, and helped prevent eleven thousand maternal deaths worldwide.[16]

These numbers tell us that we can save women's lives if we want to because we already know how. We already have the solutions, and we know where to intervene. But these numbers also tell us that women are dying needlessly in situations that are largely preventable. We have to remind ourselves that each number is a *real* woman—someone's daughter, sister, wife, mother. Every woman's life counts.

After Barack Obama won the presidency in 2008, one of his first acts was to repeal the GGR. We celebrated in our office conference rooms and toasted with champagne, but deep down we all knew it was just a temporary victory.

"Health care providers, not politicians, know what is best for their patients and families," Serra Sippel, president of the Center for Health and Gender Equity, wrote in the *Advocate*. "It is wrong for the United States to force health care providers in other countries to choose between restricting the care they can provide to patients and keeping critical funding."[17]

Until the United States *permanently* repeals this policy, women around the world will pay with their health and lives. The United States can, and must, do better. And American women must lead the way by tapping into the power of their "hysteria" to speak out for women around the world who are impacted by American policies such as the GGR.

The power of Americans, especially American women, to step in and fix the wrongs of their government is not such a radical idea. It is something that I witnessed firsthand in 2002 when the George W. Bush administration announced it was withholding $34 million in congressionally appropriated funds from the United Nations Population Fund (UNFPA), which is the UN agency for sexual and reproductive health.

The decision was made on unfounded rumors and reports that the agency was backing programs in China that included forced abortions, allegations that even the US State Department's own fact-finding team found to be false.

Enter Jane Roberts, a retired French teacher and tennis coach from Redlands, California. "A brainstorm came to me as I lay awake, anger simmering in my brain," Roberts wrote in her memoir, *34 Million Friends of the Women of the World.* "Why not, I said to myself, ask 34 million of my fellow Americans to chip in $1?"[18]

Roberts went on to devote two decades of her life to a grassroots campaign to ensure that Americans could privately support an agency that was created, ironically, at the behest of the United States in the 1960s.

Today, despite being the tireless target of GOP politicians, politics, and presidents since the 1980s, UNFPA is thriving. "We have more money than we have ever had in the history of UNFPA," said Arthur Erken, director of policy and strategy at the Population Fund.[19]

If one American woman can help curb the impact of harmful US policies on women's lives, imagine what American women could collectively do to advocate for women's health—at home and abroad.

3

A Tale as Old as Time

In researching this book, I spoke with almost one hundred women with various medical issues. All of them had had their pain dismissed by medical professionals. They were told their symptoms were the result of anxiety, depression, or stress, if not simply a figment of their imagination.

Each time, the women's pain and symptoms were found not only to be real but also indicators of serious illness. In short, no woman was imagining her illness, yet every woman was told she was.

The pattern that quickly emerged was that every woman has a sexist medical story, and every woman of color has a sexist *and* racist medical story. It was so consistent that I almost couldn't believe it. But then I realized, that is precisely the problem. Why is it so common for medical professionals not to believe women?

"Our national failure to take women seriously is a public health crisis," said Jaclyn Friedman in her essay "The Cost of Disbelieving," included in *Believe Me: How Trusting Women Can Change the*

World, the groundbreaking anthology Friedman edited with Jessica Valenti.

"Take, for example, the medical establishment's long-documented refusal to take women at our word about the symptoms we're experiencing," Friedman wrote. "Whether we're suffering from acute and chronic pain, mysterious weight loss or gain, neuromuscular conditions, or depression and anxiety, we're suspected of being melodramatic, or told that all we need is an attitude adjustment and some self-care."[1]

And it's not just women and feminists who are aware of this phenomenon. Medical professionals know it, too.

"I can't tell you how many women I've seen who have gone to see numerous doctors, only to be told their issues were stress-related or all in their heads," Dr. Fiona Gupta, a neurologist and director of wellness and health in the department of neurosurgery at the Icahn School of Medicine at Mount Sinai in New York City, told the *New York Times*. "Many of these patients were later diagnosed with serious neurological problems, like multiple sclerosis and Parkinson's disease. They knew something was wrong, but had been discounted and instructed not to trust their own intuition."[2]

Penney Cowan, founder and chief executive of the American Chronic Pain Association, agrees with Dr. Gupta. She says physicians tend to discount women's pain a lot more than they do men's. Studies back her. According to a 2014 online survey of more than 2,400 American women with a variety of chronic pain conditions, 91 percent felt that the healthcare system discriminates against female patients, and nearly half were told their pain was all in their heads.[3]

Other research has shown that clinicians are more likely to suggest psychosocial causes, such as stress, to female patients in pain even when they would order lab tests more frequently for a male patient with similar symptoms. Evidence also points to less thorough investigation of women's pain generally, especially when the cause of pain is unclear.

As with most things in healthcare, if the situation is bad for women, it's even worse for women of color, especially Black women. Studies find that compared to white patients, Black patients are 40 percent less likely to receive medication to ease acute pain and Hispanic patients are 25 percent less likely.[4]

In 2012, an analysis of twenty years of published research in the United States found that African American patients reporting pain were 22 percent less likely than white patients to get pain medication from their doctors.[5] The gap was largest when the cause was not easy to pinpoint, such as with back pain.

Another study found that African American patients reported less effective pain management than white patients.[6] One factor in this, experts say, is that some healthcare providers incorrectly believe that patients of color are more likely to abuse prescription painkillers.

"Black women, like all women across races, have a very hard time being taken seriously about their own bodies, due to a pervasive sexism," Dr. Tina Sacks, an assistant professor at UC Berkeley's School of Social Welfare and the author of *Invisible Visits: Black Middle-Class Women in the American Healthcare System*, told *Fortune*.[7] "When you compound that with racism, you have a particularly toxic mixture that Black women are facing."

Dr. Neel Shah, a Harvard Medical School professor, echoes Dr. Sacks. "[Doctors] believe Black women less when they express concerns about the symptoms they're having, particularly around pain," he said in an interview with CBS News.[8]

Perhaps the only thing more shocking than how common it is for women not to be believed about their health is how many of us opt to stay quiet about those experiences. Too many women have a medical misogyny story or a story of a near-death experience, and most of us just keep it to ourselves. It truly is a tale as old as time, and these tales must be told.

Women's health in America is often presented as a white woman's issue, but it is critical that we include the experiences of women of color because otherwise we are literally getting only half the story.

The next section focuses on case studies of women of color who had to seek medical care for serious conditions. It exposes their experiences battling aggression, bias, fear, and blatant racism in the healthcare system—and the lengths they were forced to go to prove their pain.

Before everything went dark, Asia Keyes remembered a pool of blood and the look of terror on her husband's face. Keyes is a thirty-nine-year-old African American mother of one with a master's in science and a PhD in biophysics. She has excellent health insurance. But none of this protected her from the problem that plagues Black women in the delivery room: their pain is routinely dismissed by doctors.

Keyes said that a few seconds into her scheduled C-section, she could feel the doctor cutting across her stomach. She started screaming and told her doctor, "I can feel this," but he insisted the pain was "not that bad." Keyes again repeated that she could feel her stomach being cut open.

"Even though this man was slicing me open, I tried to remain calm," Keyes told me. "I didn't want him to write me off as being hysterical, but the pain was excruciating."[9]

Keyes kept being ignored by the doctor as he continued with the procedure until she heard someone yell, "Stop!" Keyes said right after that she passed out from the pain.

"I woke up to the room being cleaned up by hospital staff," she said. "I was crying, 'What happened to the baby?' I thought maybe my baby died, and no one was there to explain anything to me—not even my doctor."

Although both Keyes and her baby survived the cesarean surgery, she said the birth of her son was so traumatic that when she got pregnant again she avoided hospitals altogether and found a midwife.

Keyes's husband, Jason, told me he was certain he was going to lose his wife and baby boy that day. He said he wanted to speak up and advocate more on behalf of his wife but worried about how the "angry Black man" stereotype could end up hurting him and his wife.

"Sometimes you just know in your bones when someone feels contempt for you based on your race," Jason said.

Amy Mason-Cooley was in so much pain that she couldn't walk. She said she felt like she was "being sliced open with a rusty handsaw." Mason-Cooley is thirty-seven years old and experiences excruciating pain from sickle cell disease, a disorder in which abnormally crescent-shaped red blood cells can get stuck in blood vessels and prevent the flow of blood and oxygen to parts of the body.

Mason-Cooley's husband rushed her to the hospital, where even after twenty-four hours, her pain still hadn't gotten any better. But her doctor decided to take her off of medications anyway, even though Mason-Cooley begged him not to. She still couldn't walk and knew her body was in crisis.

"As soon as he stopped all my medications, my blood count started dropping," she recalled to NBC News. "It dropped down low enough that they started talking about doing a transfusion."[10]

Mason-Cooley asked to be seen by another doctor, but her requests were ignored. It wasn't until other medical staff came in, believed her, and put Mason-Cooley back on her medication that, hours later, she finally stabilized. Mason-Cooley says no matter how she expresses her pain, because she is a Black woman she will always risk being dismissed.

"There's so much judgment," she said. "If you're too calm, then they say, 'Oh, you're not sick. You don't look sick.' And then if you're crying and moaning, they say you're exaggerating. I don't really know what they want from us."[11]

Mason-Cooley filed a complaint with the hospital and shared her experience in a Facebook post that went viral. Women across the country related to her story.

"Of course, having sickle cell, I know my body," Mason-Cooley told me. "Sickle cell is something you can't see. It's also predominantly found in African Americans. Studies show that 40 percent of doctors think we can tolerate so much more pain and that our pain isn't real. I have to stay alive not only for me but for the sickle cell community. So many of us die young. I read so many posts from those who suffer with the disease complain about care, being sent home, and days later, they die. No more. I do this for the youths in the sickle cell community. I want to encourage others to speak out, and don't let them kill you. Living with sickle cell is possible. It's not a death sentence . . . We have to hold those that care for us responsible."[12]

*

Fighting to breathe and struggling for air, Dr. Susan Moore was able to record herself on her phone from the hospital bed where she was being treated for COVID-19. Her video showed America how not even the status of a doctor could shield Moore, a Black woman, from negligence in the medical system.

Dr. Moore said her white doctor didn't believe she was short of breath, even though he knew he was treating a fellow licensed physician. Staff at the hospital near Indianapolis attempted to discharge her early, and her countless pleas for medication for the pain in her neck were met with sneers.

"I was crushed," Dr. Moore said in a video she posted on Facebook that went viral. "He made me feel like a drug addict. And he knew I was a physician. I don't take narcotics. I put forward and I maintain if I was white, I wouldn't have to go through that."[13]

In her video, Dr. Moore recalls her experience with the precision of a physician. Dr. Moore said doctors were ready to discharge her after only two doses of remdesivir, an antiviral drug prescribed by some physicians, and said she no longer needed the medication. She said a CT scan validated her reports of pain by showing infections and inflammation in her neck and lungs.[14]

After doctors agreed to prescribe pain medication, Dr. Moore said she waited two and a half hours to receive her initial doses, and a nurse snapped when she drew attention to the delay. She grew incensed as she recalled how the same nurse later told her he marched in a Black Lives Matter protest. Moore doesn't believe it.

"He wouldn't even know how to march, probably can't spell it," Dr. Moore said. "This is how Black people get killed. When you send them home and they don't know how to fight for themselves."[15]

Less than twelve hours after Dr. Moore returned home, her

fever and heart rate spiked. She went to a different hospital, where she died from COVID-related complications.

According to the *Washington Post* article, Indiana University Health, which operates the hospital Dr. Moore alleged mistreatment at, declined to comment on what became a very high-profile case. They said they would implement "new anti-racism, anti-bias and civility training for all team members."[16]

But Dr. Moore's story of being dismissed to death reinforces what studies have repeatedly shown: wealth, education, and insurance status do not protect Black patients from bad medical care. The outcomes are often lethal.

"We know from studies that racism doesn't stop because of your socioeconomic status or education status," Dr. Loucresie Rupert, a doctor who founded Physician Women SOAR, a group devoted to addressing racial discrimination in medicine, said in an interview to the *Washington Post*. "To see that in real time and to see the consequences, that has really shaken up a lot of the Black physicians I know."[17]

Tara Robinson, an African American woman, woke up a few weeks after her fortieth birthday in the middle of the night with a burning feeling in her chest, numbness in her jaw, nausea, and back pain.

She went to the emergency room with her husband for the first of three times that week, each time for heart attacks that Robinson and the doctors in the emergency room didn't realize she was having. "It was like an electrical circuit was not connecting at all and was firing all over the place," Robinson recalled.[18]

For a number of months leading up to that week, Robinson had been concerned about her sore neck and intermittent pain in her left arm, which her primary care physician chalked up to stress. At the ER, the doctor on call told her she was too young to have a heart attack and sent Robinson home.

She was back a few days later when the symptoms returned. The EKG didn't indicate she was having a cardiac event, but she insisted the hospital keep her overnight. Doctors wanted to send her home because her symptoms did not appear to be life-threatening, but she knew she had to listen to her body, which was telling her something was very wrong.

The hospital discharged Robinson the next morning without any instructions. Then came the third visit, another overnight stay, and a morning discharge. Just hours later, at 4:00 p.m., Robinson was rushed to the hospital with a massive heart attack, a 99 percent blockage in her main artery. Doctors inserted a stent to reestablish the blood flow.[19]

"I tell women that you're the best advocate for your health," Robinson said.[20] "Nobody knows your body like you know it."

Robinson later discovered that heart disease runs in her family. Her experience prompted her to become a spokesperson for the Go Red for Women campaign, the American Heart Association's signature women's initiative.

"We have to start as women to put ourselves first and make a commitment to living a healthier lifestyle," she said.[21]

When author, sociologist, and professor Tressie McMillan Cottom started bleeding at her obstetrician's office, she was four months pregnant. Her doctor told her it was probably because she was "just too fat,"[22] the spotting was normal, and sent her home. Cottom recalls how later that night, her butt started hurting. After speaking to her mother, she called the nurse, who asked her if it was her back that was hurting.

"I said no," Cottom wrote. "It was my butt that hurt. The nurse said it was probably constipation. I should try to go to the bathroom. I tried that for all the next day and part of another. By the end of three days, my butt still hurt and I had not slept more than fifteen minutes straight in almost seventy hours."[23]

Cottom finally went to the hospital, where medical staff asked again if it was her back, suggested she ate something bad, and then finally decided to do an ultrasound.

"The image showed three babies, only I was pregnant with one," Cottom said. "The other two were tumors, larger than the baby. The doctor turned to me and said, 'If you make it through the night without going into preterm labor, I'd be surprised.' With that, he walked out and I was checked into the maternity ward. Eventually a night nurse mentioned that I had been in labor for three days. 'You should have said something,' she scolded me."[24]

After several days of labor pains that no one ever diagnosed, Cottom said she could not hold off labor anymore. She recalled how she was wheeled into a delivery operating room, where she slipped in and out of consciousness.

"At one point I awoke and screamed, 'Motherfucker.' The nurse told me to watch my language. I begged for an epidural. After three eternities an anesthesiologist arrived. He glared at me and said that if I wasn't quiet he would leave and I would not get any pain relief . . . I tried desperately to be still and quiet so he would not leave me there that way. Thirty seconds after the injection, I passed out before my head hit the pillow."[25]

When Cottom woke up, she said she was pushing and then her daughter was born. The baby died soon afterward.

"The nurse wheeled me out of the operating room to take me back to recovery," Cottom wrote. "I held my baby the whole way, because apparently that is what is done. After making plans for how we would handle her remains, the nurse turned to me and said, 'Just so you know, there was nothing we could have done, because you did not tell us you were in labor.'"[26]

Cottom says that like millions of women of color, especially Black women, the "healthcare machine could not imagine me as competent and so it neglected and ignored me until I was incompetent." She wrote that when the medical profession systematically denies the existence of Black women's pain, underdiagnoses it, refuses to alleviate or treat it, "healthcare marks us as incompetent bureaucratic subjects. Then it serves us accordingly."[27]

What do the experiences of Asia Keyes, Dr. Susan Moore, Amy Mason-Cooley, Tara Robinson, and Tressie McMillan Cottom tell us? That Black women in America should expect to receive the lowest quality care from the medical establishment due to racism and discrimination. And that is putting it mildly.

In 2020, both the *New England Journal of Medicine* and *The Lancet*,[28] two of the world's oldest medical journals, identified racism in America as a public health crisis, confirming what many women of color already know: we are objectified, ignored, and violently handled in medical settings.[29]

"I think Black life in general, and Black female (cis and trans) lives in particular, are devalued in the United States," Dr. Sacks told me. "This extends to other women of color, disabled women, and immigrant women. . . . There are so many structural barriers to health and wellness, including mental well-being. The American healthcare system is so fragmented, and it's so hard to get good care unless you have a lot of money, and even then there are many challenges. All of these things create a perfect storm."[30]

We see this play out in Keyes's experience. Despite her various educational degrees, she was still treated no better than an animal when she was giving birth. The statistic that Black mothers are three times, or 243 percent, more likely to die from pregnancy-related issues than white mothers[31] leads to the racist misconception that Black women are low-income, uneducated, and unable to advocate for themselves.

But in reality, many of the women behind these alarming numbers are highly educated and more than capable of advocating for themselves. In fact, the Centers for Disease Control and Prevention (CDC) says the pregnancy-related Black mortality ratio is actually *higher* among women with a college degree: educated Black women are 5.2 times more likely to die due to pregnancy-related complications than their similarly educated white counterparts.[32]

"Many of the women I interviewed would have that inkling that they weren't getting the same care as their white counterparts, but there really is no way to know for sure, because you are only one person, and you don't really have a control group," Dr. Sacks said.[33] "And part of the challenge of that experience is the anxiety about whether or not it is true. 'Can I trust my own perceptions? And what can I do about it?'"

Dr. Sacks tells her own story of how at the start of her career, when she worked for the CDC, she and her Black female colleagues would make it a point to wear their government IDs when going to the doctor for checkups.

It was a way to "telegraph" that they were professionals who understood medical terminology and had good health insurance, all so medical staff would take them seriously. "In other words, we were playing against a type," Sacks wrote in her book.

Asia Keyes's story of being cut open during her C-section without adequate pain medication shows that multiple degrees won't save Black women when it comes to their health. Their education cannot protect them from implicit biases that reduce women of color to the color of our skin.

We see this again in Dr. Susan Moore's video, which reminded Americans how the coronavirus pandemic is ravaging African American and other communities of color, while simultaneously exposing rampant racism in the country's healthcare system.

Tara Robinson's near-fatal experience shows us how crucial it is to be armed with information. In her case, it wasn't her doctors but Robinson herself who saved her own life by knowing how stereotypes and racism can dismiss women to death. Robinson was smart to be informed with the stats, but she was lucky she was able to get the critical care she needed. Studies show that when a Black woman speaks up to advocate for herself, she is often marked as "angry" and "combative" by medical staff. And doctors know it, too.

4

Invisible Conditions

When Shereen Abdel-Nabi found her vaginal cyst had grown exponentially, she immediately went to her ob-gyn. After diagnosing it as a Bartholin cyst, her OB proceeded to drain it at her office, a procedure Abdel-Nabi calls "worse than childbirth."[1] When she wound up at the ER and asked for pain medication, she was told the hospital was "trying really hard not to give those out anymore."

After the appointment, Abdel-Nabi proceeded to take her nine-year-old son to soccer practice because, as she honestly points out, that's what moms do. "You leave work, have a traumatic procedure, but make it home in time for soccer practice," Abdel-Nabi said.

By the following morning, her pain was so unbearable that she wound up in the emergency room. Unlike her OB visit, the ER doctor gave her a hydromorphine drip before beginning what Abdel-Nabi describes as a procedure from the Dark Ages.

"I was only given the drip because I was so traumatized by

the doctor's office visit, and the pain I had been in, that I basically begged her to do something more than 'numb the area,'" Abdel-Nabi recalled. "She reluctantly gave it to me as if she was doing me some sort of favor."

Abdel-Nabi said she was stuck in a freezing-cold trauma room because that's what was available. "The doctor made me sit on an upside-down bedpan as she sliced me some more," Abdel-Nabi said. "I screamed and cried so loud that the Jamaican nurse assigned to her had to leave the room for it because she couldn't stand being in there."

The following week, Abdel-Nabi returned to her OB for a follow-up, as per the ER doctor, only to be told her catheter wasn't placed in a way that would properly drain the cyst.

"The catheter was placed in such a way that I basically had an open wound for several days," Abdel-Nabi recalled. "I couldn't sit or lay down properly because it was literally jutting out of me—and it was all for naught."

Abdel-Nabi pleaded with her doctor to be put under anesthesia because she could not mentally or physically handle another "barbaric" procedure. Although the cyst was successfully drained in the OR, Abdel-Nabi says she remains traumatized by the experience.

"My overwhelming feeling is that my pain was dismissed at every stage," Abdel-Nabi said. "The only person who took my pain seriously was the Jamaican nurse, and she couldn't even stand to be in the room. This was a procedure that was originally done in an operating room. If I had been a man, this would have been a completely different medical experience. How are we still subjecting women to this kind of treatment in the twenty-first century?"

Abdel-Nabi says her experience highlights how women die because some "certainly male doctor" decided that a procedure that should be done under full anesthesia in an OR can be done at the end of the day in a doctor's office—or in whatever available room the ER can find you when they're busy.

"And this is a best-case scenario," Abdel-Nabi said. "This is with great health insurance and access to the best care. It's unacceptable."

When author, model, *Top Chef* TV host, and cofounder of the Endometriosis Foundation of America Padma Lakshmi was finally diagnosed and treated for endometriosis, she was relieved. But then she got angry.

"I was diagnosed at thirty-six after suffering every month since the age of thirteen with so much heavy bleeding, cramps, nausea, backaches, and digestive issues that I was stuck in bed one week out of every month when my period came," Lakshmi said in a speech at the Massachusetts Institute of Technology (MIT) Center for Gynepathology Research. "One week a month—three months a year—for twenty-three years. That's five years and nine months of my life that I was bedridden."[2]

Before finally getting a diagnosis in 2006, none of the gynecologists Lakshmi consulted had ever mentioned the disease endometriosis to her. For more than two decades, Lakshmi struggled to manage the chronic pain that arrived in tandem with her monthly period.

Like so many young girls, she was told that painful cramps—even severe ones—were part of the "burden of being a female."[3] But over the years, the pain steadily increased, worsening month by month and year after year.

Eventually, Lakshmi ended up in bed for days at a time, desperately trying to alleviate the pain with hot-water bottles and heating pads. She drank herbal teas and downed over-the-counter or prescription pain relievers such as Tylenol. When the pain was unbearable, she took stronger pain medication such as codeine or Vicodin. Lakshmi says she also suffered from a lot of digestive issues.

"Around my period, I'd get constipated and feel nauseous," she said, in an interview with *Practical Pain Management* (*PPM*).[4] She had headaches, backaches, and shooting pains down her leg.

Lakshmi was told by doctors that she had a "low threshold for pain" and that she should just get used to it because there was nothing that could be done.

"Well, it turns out I have a really high threshold for pain," Lakshmi said.[5] "Most women do; we have to. And not just for childbirth. I should have been diagnosed, treated, and relieved for my symptoms twenty years ago. Most women with endo don't get properly diagnosed for a full decade."

In 2006, during a photo shoot for her second cookbook, Lakshmi says she began to bleed heavily in mid-cycle. Aware of her ongoing menstrual issues, her doctor recommended she see the laparoscopic surgeon and endometriosis specialist Dr. Tamer Seckin. That appointment and the treatment that followed changed Lakshmi's life.

Dr. Seckin told Lakshmi he believed she had severe endometriosis, and during surgery, he found multiple endometriosis implants and lesions in Lakshmi.

"My kidneys were in stents, I had stitches on four major organs," Lakshmi wrote in her memoir. "Of the nineteen biopsies performed, seventeen came back positive as deeply infiltrating endometriosis tissue," she says.[6]

Dr. Seckin also informed her that during a previous surgery, part of her left ovary had been removed, a "detail" the prior surgeon had neglected to share with her.

Today, Lakshmi is doing much better but endometriosis still "rears its ugly head from time to time."

"I have stage IV endometriosis," Lakshmi said in the interview with *PPM*. "There's treatment but no cure for it. I still have some issues now, but they are nowhere near where they were. I'm very lucky that I was able to get the surgeries and the help that I needed."[7]

The anger she felt toward the disease and how it impacted her life is also getting better.

"I don't get angry anymore, because I'm in good company," she told PPM.[8] "Now I just want to make sure that the next generation of young girls and women don't go through what I did and do. I believe that we have the technology and brain power to find a cure."

Alicia Lopez, a Latina woman with a chronic-pain condition, says many of the doctors she encountered after she left her life in the city were more willing to believe that she was a drug addict seeking opioids than a PhD candidate.

Lopez was diagnosed with lupus when she was a graduate student, but after she moved to Charlottesville, Virginia, to finish her dissertation, she was frequently accused of feeding a drug habit. Doctors refused to treat her, and pharmacists regularly questioned her.

For an entire year, Lopez said she was unable to find adequate care to manage or treat her pain. This was after numerous calls to Lopez's doctors in Virginia by specialists she had seen previously.

Everything came to a head one night when, after entering the emergency room and asking to be admitted, Lopez was held in a room for *six* hours as doctor after doctor came in and attempted to convince her that she did not have lupus and that she did not need to be in the hospital.

It was only at hour seven, after Lopez was crying hysterically, yelling at doctors and holding hands with an empathetic nurse, that a new doctor came on rotation. "He looked at me once and admitted me without any questions," Lopez said.[9]

Once admitted, doctors were able to easily treat the inflammation and symptoms causing Lopez's excruciating pain, a lupus trademark.

While Lopez says she will forever be grateful for the doctor who believed her and showed her compassion when no one else did, she points out that women of color should not have to depend on their random luck of being seen by a good doctor to get adequate healthcare.

"Women of color should not have to prove the legitimacy of their illnesses in order to get treatment," Lopez said. "Perhaps this can only happen with the dismantling of racism, but for the sake of women who suffer from chronic pain, I hope our time comes sooner."[10]

Catherine Rakowski was twenty-nine years old when she was completing a master's degree in psychology in New York. "My research was, ironically, based purely in empathy," she recalled. "I helped run the largest study at the time on coupled gay men, and my thesis related to their desire and mental health around becoming parents. I myself donated eggs to a gay couple who had sought a half-Asian donor."[11]

Rakowski said that in retrospect, the misogyny began with the fertility clinic. "Egg donation builds in the bias, because it's women who produce eggs, and the discomfort and potential pain can only be physically understood by women," she said.[12]

HCG is the pregnancy hormone; it's what doctors test for to determine whether a woman is pregnant. To release the excess eggs, a doctor administers a large shot of HCG, and the eggs are retrieved twelve hours later. But the effects of the HCG shot have a seven-day half-life, which no one had told Rakowski.

"Five days after my extraordinarily successful egg retrieval (thirty-one eggs in a single cycle), I arrived at the hospital with ovarian hyperstimulation—a term no one had introduced to me at the time," she said. "I hadn't eaten in about thirty-six hours, I had been vomiting for as long, and I'd barely been able to urinate. My best friend says I was gray. My torso was distended and disfigured. I had been unable to speak for a few hours because my pain was so intense."[13]

Rakowski said she was given fluids and antinausea medication by IV, and doctors took blood and ran tests, including a pregnancy test. She said she doesn't know how she mustered the strength and articulation to tell her story to triage, to nurses, to doctor after doctor.

"I saw five doctors (all male) and twelve nurses (mostly female) throughout my overnight stay," Rakowski said. "I'll never forget the moment two white male doctors continued to ask me questions without pausing as I vomited bile into a tray."

Her pregnancy test came back, and they told her she was pregnant. "I explained myself well, consistently, and accurately," Rakowski said. "And yet, they sent me home in far worse shape than I arrived."

Rakowski later learned that her excruciating pain was from the fluid pressuring her organs, which was impeding her metabolism and digestion. "I could have died from liver failure that night," she said. She eventually had seven liters of fluid (fifteen pounds!) drained out of her abdomen back at the fertility clinic.

"I entered the process feeling empowered and like an equal stakeholder," Rakowski said. "I was a fully-fledged adult with a great education and vocabulary to advocate for myself. I left feeling like a commodity whose pain and risk were afterthoughts. (While I was still recovering, the clinic called to ask if I would donate again. Aghast, I declined.) All the doctors at the fertility clinic were men. I knew there was some unknown risk, but I was not fairly informed. I had so much in my favor. But ultimately I was a woman dealing with men who didn't inform me and then didn't believe me."

Rakowski said if she were to do it again, she would want to know more. "I would seek a clinic or agency that prides itself in its treatment of donors, that offered conversations with previous donors," she said. "Would I want to speak with a female physician? Maybe, but I'm not convinced that would have made much of a difference. Internalized misogyny is alive and well in medicine and in every industry."

When Amal Abdel-Rahman checked in to her hospital, as an Arab American and Muslim woman, she felt early on that her opinions didn't matter to the ob-gyn team that was overseeing her delivery.

When Abdel-Rahman asked for an epidural, the anesthesiologist told her she'd have to prove she was in enough pain first. "I had to perform labor pain to his expectations before he would authorize the epidural," Abdel-Rahman said.[14]

When an epidural was finally approved, Abdel-Rahman was surprised it wasn't the anesthesiologist who gave it to her but a student he'd delegated to do the task. Abdel-Rahman said the student missed three times, ultimately stabbing her in the spine a total of four times before the medication was delivered. The student then set the epidural for only forty minutes, saying she wanted it to wear off before Abdel-Rahman went into labor.

"After the epidural wore off, I was in horrific pain," Abdel-Rahman recalled.[15] "I was screaming, having trouble breathing, and panicking. A nurse came in the room and told me to 'shut up' because I was scaring other patients. By the time I was ready to deliver, I'd been laboring med-free for about an hour and a half."

What followed were third-degree tears after the medical team failed to give Abdel-Rahman an episiotomy, something she'd had with her first baby. The nursing staff also cleaned her baby shortly after delivery but left Abdel-Rahman lying in sheets soaked with blood and fluids for more than an hour after she gave birth.

"Giving birth is supposed to be such an empowering moment in a woman's life, but the medical staff treated me like an animal," Abdel-Rahman said. "I had to perform for my pain to be believed in the middle of childbirth. It was humiliating. But how do I prove I was treated as subhuman because I am a Brown, Middle Eastern woman?"

The stories of Abdel-Nabi, Lakshmi, Lopez, Rakowski, and Abdel-Rahman show us not only how common it is for women's pain not to be taken seriously, but also how medical professionals expect women to just accept their pain as a "normal" part of being a woman. It's almost as though they think suffering and womanhood go hand in hand.

Feminist writer Maya Dusenbery, author of *Doing Harm: The Truth about How Bad Medicine and Lazy Science Leave Women Dismissed,*

Misdiagnosed, and Sick, is a white woman who never thought much about her health until she developed rheumatoid arthritis at the age of twenty-seven.

Dusenbery's symptoms began a couple of weeks after a bad bout of the flu. She woke up one morning, and her knuckles and hands were painful and stiff. Over the course of the next few months, the stiffness worsened, spreading from her hands to her ankles and toes to her knees, and eventually to her shoulders and elbows as well.[16]

Rheumatoid arthritis is an autoimmune disease in which the immune system starts attacking the lining of the joints. Dusenbery was lucky—she went to the right doctor and got diagnosed quickly and accurately, but her story does not end there.

The more she spoke with other women with autoimmune or other chronic-pain conditions, the more Dusenbery realized how unusual and difficult getting a diagnosis is. Most women she spoke with complained of doctors not having autoimmune diseases on their radar, or being dismissed without follow-ups, or being told, yet again, that their pain was all in their heads.

"I wanted to sort of understand what was happening to my own body, and as I learned more about autoimmune diseases was very struck by the fact that they are very common," Dusenbery explained in an interview to National Public Radio (NPR).[17]

Being a feminist journalist and editor of Feministing.com, Dusenbery says it wasn't rocket science for her to make the connection between the fact that three-quarters of people with autoimmune diseases are women and the amount of time it takes to get an accurate diagnosis. She found that on average, female patients take three and a half years, and see at least five doctors, before getting a diagnosis.

"It's easy to label a woman as a chronic complainer and be dismissive of her pain rather than assume she has a medical disorder," Dusenbery said, adding that she thinks medicine hasn't really moved on from hysteria and that the concept has just been rebranded for the modern era.[18]

"In recent decades, unexplained symptoms that previous generations would have called 'hysteria' have just gotten new labels: terms like 'psychogenic,' 'functional' or 'medically unexplained symptoms,'" Dusenbery pointed out. "By and large, medicine has held on to the idea that any physical symptoms that cannot currently be explained physiologically can, by default, be attributed to the psyche. This idea is dangerous for all patients, and it continues to particularly harm women, who frequently encounter health care providers who say or imply that their symptoms are 'all in their heads.'"[19]

What do all these women's stories tell us, from Asia Keyes to Shereen Abdel-Nabi to Tara Robinson to Padma Lakshmi to Dr. Susan Moore to Maya Dusenbery? They tell us that women's pain is not taken as seriously as men's, and that the problem is systemic. It's not just a matter of a few sexist doctors but rather a whole system that has historically marginalized women and minimized our suffering.

The majority of doctors nationwide are white, and research suggests they often underestimate the pain level of minority patients.[20] A 2016 University of Virginia study even found that half of the hundreds of white medical students and residents surveyed believe at least one myth about alleged racial differences related to pain— such as believing that the nerve endings of Black people are less sensitive than those of white people. The study found that those who believed this and other racist myths were more likely to rate a Black patient as having less pain—and to undertreat.[21]

Associate news editor of the *Guardian* newspaper and author of *Pain and Prejudice* Gabrielle Jackson says her pain from endometriosis made life unbearable. After more than a decade of writing herself off as a hypochondriac, Jackson decided to take matters into her own hands.[22]

During the course of her research, Jackson found that not believing women about their pain was worse than she imagined. She wrote that while studies show women wait longer for pain medication than men and are more likely to have their physical symptoms ascribed to mental health issues, what was among the most shocking to Jackson was learning about the number of women who live with constant pain.[23]

"I discovered that there are 10 chronic pain conditions that predominantly affect women which have very similar symptoms; and that once a person has one, they're more likely to accumulate others," Jackson said in a *Guardian* article.[24]

She believes that the medical community has known for a century that women are living in constant pain but have done nothing about it.

"I wrote this book because too many women are in pain, and that pain is not taken seriously," Jackson wrote. "It is at once expected and denied. This deprives us of our full humanity. We deserve better."[25]

When did things get so bad for women? Were we always viewed as irrational and untrustworthy creatures when it came to our health? Apparently, yes.

In ancient times, the womb was believed to be the root of all the medical problems experienced by women, and there is roughly four thousand years of historical evidence pointing to people actually believing all this. An Egyptian papyrus dating from about 1900

BCE includes recipes for medicines to coax a "wandering uterus" back to its proper place in the body.[26]

We know Greek philosopher Hippocrates famously believed that the uterus was a "free-floating" animal and that his equally sexist peer Plato shared the idea. A Hippocratic medical text from the fifth century BCE puts it more bluntly by stating that "the womb is the origin of all diseases in women." In the Middle Ages, women's "hysterical symptoms" were attributed to the retention of "sexual fluid."[27]

By the late 1800s, medical and scientific interest in hysteria reached a fever pitch, and it soon became a blanket term for various "female issues," from fainting to sleeplessness to irritability to nervousness, and (my personal favorite) "a tendency to cause trouble for others."[28]

French neurologist Jean-Martin Charcot proposed that hysteria was a nerve disease similar to multiple sclerosis and not unique to women. Soon after, Sigmund Freud came along to argue that hysteria was rooted in "unconscious conflicts" that converted themselves into bodily symptoms. He coined this "conversion hysteria."[29]

While these theories may vary, one aspect remains consistent: men have been wrongly labeling and dismissing women as "hysterical" since the dawn of time—literally from the ancient Egyptians to the Greeks to Freud. It makes you wonder if these men even believed these theories themselves, or whether their egos were just too big to admit what they simply didn't know.

"The historical hysteria discourse was most often endorsed when discussing 'difficult' women, referring to those for whom treatment was not helpful or who held a perception of their disease alternative to their clinician," Dr. Kate Young, a research fellow at the School of Public Health and Preventive Medicine at Monash University in Melbourne, Australia, wrote in the journal *Feminism*

& Psychology. "Rather than acknowledge the limitations of medical knowledge, medicine expected women to take control (with their minds) of their disease (in their body) by accepting their illness, making 'lifestyle' changes and conforming to their gendered social roles of wife and mother," Young said. "Moralising discourses surround those who rebel; they are represented as irrational and irresponsible, the safety net for medicine when it cannot fulfil its claim to control the body."[30]

Young points out that, historically, "men have made the medical science about women and their bodies," and that knowledge has been constructed to reinforce theories surrounding women and hysteria.[31]

So how can women take our power back? If not believing women has been standard for so long, what alternative can we offer the medical community? Instead of the knee-jerk reaction of dismissing women's voices, why don't doctors and medical professionals start to *believe* women? Let us start there—by trusting women and giving them the benefit of the doubt.

Doctors and medical professionals must stop dismissing women's real pain and physical symptoms and brushing us off as emotionally unstable. It has been going on for too long, and too many women have paid with their lives. Women, especially women of color, are dismissed, sometimes to death. After all this time, there should be serious, even legal, consequences for gaslighting women about our health.

Women should act *more*, not less, "hysterical" when it comes to our well-being, and that begins by telling our stories loudly. Women should embrace the power of hysteria and rethink it as a positive response—a way to speak our voice instead of staying silent. Instead of doubting our instincts, let's start sharing our stories.

"I think when you start talking about these really frustrating, disrespectful experiences in the medical system, women see that they're not alone, that it's not just them, that they share these experiences with a lot of other women," Dusenbery said in an interview with NPR. "And I think that a sort of storytelling about this can really be powerful in just sort of putting it on the radar and exposing the extent of the problem."[32]

Interviewing women and hearing their stories always brings me back to my own traumatic story. I think about what happened to me as I tried to bring my first child into the world, how I wish I had stood up to that doctor who completely disregarded my humanity. I am blessed that both my baby girl and I made it out alive, but the trauma of how I was treated very much remains.

I think about that doctor every day, and I am filled with rage. I think about how he demanded I get on the operating table myself, without any assistance from the nurses who had rolled me to the OR on a stretcher. I think about how, as I lay on that operating table, a pregnant woman in labor, shaking from a severe fever, surrounded by medical staff preparing for my emergency C-section surgery, I was repeatedly ignored when I asked for blankets. Even now, I can feel the cold of the metal table.

Nine years later, I am still absorbing the shock of my birth story, even as I write this book. Did my doctor treat me the way he did because I was just some Brown woman in his operating theater? Would he have behaved that way if my skin were white?

To be honest, I didn't really think about the racial implications of my story until I began working on this book, but it's something I harbor deep within. Whenever I force myself to think back and analyze harder, the truth is, I am filled with more shame than rage. I feel embarrassed about how I allowed myself to be handled.

I do take some comfort in the fact that, after I was discharged, I reported the doctor to the president of the hospital. As a result, he was removed from the hospital board and banned from working late-night shifts. The hospital also refunded me the anesthesia costs. But I wish I had taken legal action. The truth is, so soon after becoming a new mom, I had neither the physical nor emotional strength.

Like so many women, I thought childbirth was going to be the most empowering experience of my life, and I was ready for it to be just that. Instead, a Bangladeshi girl almost died giving birth in America. I hate that I had this experience, and I hate having to tell such a story.

But it is a story that must be told. Women, especially women of color, must come forth with our experiences of sexism *and* racism in healthcare because no one else will tell them for us. And we shouldn't want them to. Our stories are our power, and if we don't trust ourselves to tell them, no one else will believe us.

5

We Don't Know
What We Don't Know

When I was eight years old, my aunt Tazreen Ahmed got into a near-fatal car accident. My *khala* (Bengali for "maternal aunt") and her Lebanese boyfriend, George, were out partying with friends when they decided to go on a late-night drive on Dhaka's infamous Airport Road.

In the 1980s, the capital of Bangladesh was not nearly as "developed" as it is today, and there were only a few really big, wide roads. Airport Road was one of the largest roads in the city. With no white or yellow painted lanes, this massive avenue started at one end of town and took you all the way to the national airport. It was notorious for drunk driving–related car crashes, almost always involving intoxicated truckers on long cross-country routes.

When they found the car of my *khala* and her friends, it was totaled. The authorities had searched all the following day for my *khala*'s body. They finally found her, trapped under the back seat of the destroyed car. It was a miracle she survived.

But from the moment she got to the hospital, her treatment

was a nightmare. The hospital was out of even the most basic supplies. I remember my mother sending our driver out to buy Savlon (a local antiseptic) and cotton balls. It took so long for the doctor to show up at the emergency room that my mom and her other sisters used parts of their saris for slings for my *khala*'s broken arms and legs.

The experience of watching her fighting for her life in that hospital was traumatic. I remember pleading with my parents to fly my aunt out of the country. "Can't we pay to take her to America?" I begged. It made me even more aware of the massive gaps in the kind of medical care Bangladeshis had access to, and I hated the unfairness of it.

Growing up in Bangladesh, whenever we heard someone was going to the States for an operation or treatment, we believed they were going to get the best medical care possible. I considered American doctors and hospitals the gold standard.

It wasn't until my own birth experience that I became aware of America's shocking maternal mortality numbers, the highest among industrialized nations. Despite working as a feminist policy analyst at that time with a portfolio largely focused on women's reproductive health and rights, I had no idea that I should be concerned about the state of maternal health in the richest, most scientifically advanced country on earth.

Almost becoming a maternal mortality statistic myself opened my eyes to how dangerous going to a hospital as a woman in America can be. It also made me see that if you're a woman of color, you are at a higher risk of being dismissed to death.

In addition to not being believed about their pain, women also face another glaring issue—a serious lack of clinical trials and information on women's health. Both Maya Dusenbery and Gabrielle

Jackson point to this scientific and problematic gender gap in their books.

Dusenbery identifies two problems women face in the medical system. The first she calls the "trust gap," the tendency not to trust women and to dismiss their unexplained symptoms; to normalize, minimize, or attribute them to psychological causes. The second is what she calls the "knowledge gap," the fact that much less is known about women's bodies, and that diseases may manifest themselves in us differently than they do in men.[1]

Jackson echoed Dusenbery, telling me in an interview that the thing that stunned her most during the course of her research was how little medicine actually knows about female biology.

"Almost everything we know about human health comes from the study of male humans, male animals, and even male cell lines," Jackson said. "I was absolutely gobsmacked when I realised the full extent of our omission from medical science. It's no wonder doctors dismiss us—they literally know very little about us! Complaints that women make more than men have been put down to 'hysteria' or 'anxiety' for millennia, not because women are innately unstable or unable to cope but because medicine has never bothered to investigate the symptoms! I'm still shocked by this, every day."[2]

Iranian American writer and mental health advocate Melody Moezzi says that the healthcare system was not built with women, especially women of color, in mind.

"The American healthcare system is no different than any other American system," Moezzi told me in an interview. "It is a system that was designed to perpetuate broader societal values and biases, including racism, sexism, heteronormativity . . . It is a system intended to benefit some over others, because—like the American criminal justice and the educational systems—the American healthcare system does not value all lives equally . . . It is a system that values white, male, wealthy, straight, cisgender, able-bodied, neurotypical individuals above all others."[3]

All women should be shocked about the systematic exclusion of women from testing and clinical trials—and justifiably so. Between the 1970s and 1990s, both the National Institutes of Health (NIH) and the Food and Drug Administration (FDA), along with other regulators, had a policy that ruled out women of so-called childbearing potential from early-stage drug trials.[4] The result was that *all women* were excluded from trials, regardless of their age, gender status, sexual orientation, or wish or ability to bear children.[5] The general justification for excluding women, and making the male body the default, was that males are cheaper to study because their hormonal systems are simpler.[6]

"We literally know less about every aspect of female biology compared to male biology," Dr. Janine Austin Clayton, an associate director for women's health research at the United States National Institutes of Health, told the *Guardian* in November 2019.[7]

The good news is that women mobilized after finding out about their widespread and systematic exclusion. During the 1980s, a group of American female scientists formed the Society for Women's Health Research to campaign for better health research in women. They teamed up with members of Congress to draw attention to the serious inconsistencies in medical research and the impact they have on women's health.[8] Their findings were astounding.

For example, in the 1960s, researchers conducted the first trial to look at whether hormonal supplementation was an effective preventive treatment for women—but then enrolled 8,341 men and no women.[9] The Physicians' Health Study from 1982 analyzed the effect of a daily aspirin on heart disease, but tested 22,071 men and no women.[10] There was a 1986 pilot study from New York City's Rockefeller University exploring how obesity impacts breast and uterine cancer that also failed to include women in the studies—even though men don't have uteruses.[11] It goes on and on.

And things aren't much better today, as women continue to be underrepresented in studies. The NIH didn't open an Office of Research on Women's Health until 1990, when the gynecological symptoms of AIDS began to show up,[12] sending a clear message that trials needed to include and focus on women.

Finally in 1993, the FDA and the NIH mandated the inclusion of women in clinical trials, officially requiring all federally funded clinical research to prioritize the inclusion of "women and under-served racial and ethnic groups."[13] But it still took until 2014 for the NIH to acknowledge the widespread issue of male bias in pre-clinical trials.[14] And it wasn't until 2016 that they mandated that the studies had to include women in order to be granted research money.[15]

That science and medicine have a gender problem, and that it affects what is studied, is an understatement. For example, even though 70 percent of patients impacted by chronic pain are women, 80 percent of pain studies continue to be on men or male mice.[16]

In addition to this gender problem, the medical world's diversity problem is not any better. Between 1993 and 2013, less than 2 percent of cancer studies included enough racial and ethnic group participants to report relevant results.[17] Most clinical research includes participants who are still overwhelmingly white, non-Hispanic, and, until recently, male. More than 80 percent of genome-wide studies, which are related to DNA biology, have been conducted among individuals of European descent, and Hispanics represent only 0.54 percent of participants.[18]

"When it comes to clinical trials funded by pharmaceutical companies, the FDA encourages but does not require diversity in clinical trials," Diana Zuckerman, president of the National Center for Health Research and a scientist herself, told *Fortune* magazine.[19] She points out that the FDA regularly approves drugs and devices for all adults—even if they were primarily studied only on white male adults.

Again, this has serious—and potentially lethal—implications for women's health. A recent example is how differently Ambien and other prescription sleeping pills affect men and women. Because women metabolize the drug more slowly than men, women can still be too drowsy to operate a vehicle even as long as eight hours after taking it. The FDA had to go back and cut the recommended dosage for women in half after finding this out in 2018.[20]

In 2020, a team of experts from Northwestern University and Smith College decided to see whether women were still being excluded from biomedical research based on concerns that female hormonal variations complicated findings. They examined more than seven hundred scientific journal articles published in 2019, from nine fields, and found that compared to 2009, the number of studies that included females had increased from 28 percent to 49 percent.[21]

But despite that one bright spot, in eight of the nine fields studied, the proportion of studies that analyzed study results by sex generally had not improved. And in pharmacology, the trend was decreasing from 33 percent to 29 percent.[22]

This lack of testing also has a serious impact on how women are diagnosed. One of the most significant examples of how science dismisses women can be seen with heart disease. Although heart disease and stroke are the leading causes of death for women in America, we are only now facing the fact that for thirty-five years, heart disease was really studied only in men.[23]

The increased attention on how women's heart disease symptoms differ from men's has led medical professionals to conclude that women are indeed more likely to have "atypical" symptoms, a.k.a. "unlike men's." For example, for women it is common during heart attacks to experience pain in the neck or shoulder and to feel nauseated, fatigued, and light-headed. These are very different from the sharp chest pains men experience in real life as well as in the movies.

Partly as a result of these differences in symptoms—which are still not always recognized by healthcare providers—women, especially younger women, are more likely to be turned away when they're having a heart attack. One study found that women under the age of fifty-five are *seven times* more likely than the average patient to be misdiagnosed and sent home mid–heart attack.[24]

Yet again, the numbers for women of color are much worse. Black women have a higher chance of dying from heart disease and at a younger age than white women. About 49 percent of African American women over age twenty have some type of cardiac infarction, and more than 60 percent of Black women are living with some form of the condition.[25]

You would think that by now, knowing what we know, diversification by race and gender would be mandated in all clinical trials. But even after watching the massive gendered impact of COVID-19 unfold in 2020, women are still systematically excluded from studies. This time, it is for the most anticipated vaccine of our lifetime—the COVID vaccine.

Even though women make up three-quarters of healthcare

workers, including more than 85 percent of nurses, and women of childbearing age making up approximately 70 percent of frontline workers, pregnant women are not being included in vaccine trials.[26] This is despite calls from medical experts, doctors, medical journals, and pregnant women themselves.

Experts know that pregnant women are at higher risk for getting COVID. In fact, the MMWR (Morbidity and Mortality Weekly Report) from the Centers for Disease Control and Prevention estimated that pregnant women are at *three times* higher risk for being admitted into an ICU or requiring a ventilator if they get COVID.[27]

The risk of dying from the coronavirus is also 70 percent higher for pregnant women, and according to a 2020 study by the CDC, expectant women of color are more at risk for contracting COVID.[28] The maternal death rate for Black mothers was already double the rate of white mothers, pre-pandemic. Nationally, Black and Latina women are also more likely to be affected by COVID during pregnancy than their white peers.[29]

How can we say we have a vaccine for everyone until we have a vaccine for our frontline workers, 70 percent of whom are women of childbearing age? We cannot. It should be a priority to give frontline workers who are pregnant, might be pregnant, or are thinking about getting pregnant the information they need to make the best and safest possible decision for themselves. So why aren't they receiving it?

"There are actually very few medications, for example, that are approved in pregnancy because it's easier, basically," Denise Jamieson, chair of the Department of Gynecology and Obstetrics at Emory University School of Medicine, and part of the American College of Obstetricians and Gynecologists' working group on

COVID-19, said in an interview with NPR. She said pregnant women are systematically excluded from most clinical trials in the United States because it makes running the trials less complicated. "It's easier to exclude pregnant women because when you include pregnant women, you have to be concerned about both the woman's health as well as the development of the fetus and baby."[30]

Jamieson says that even though pregnant women have been given vaccines for decades with few issues, live viral vaccines are generally not given in pregnancy because "there's theoretical risk that the live virus could be passed and it infects the fetus."[31]

To me, this whole "We must protect pregnant women from vaccines for the sake of the baby" answer reminds me of society's larger issue with trusting women with their bodies. In the early weeks of the historic COVID vaccine rollout in December 2020, I appeared on MSNBC's *Morning Joe*, advocating for pregnant women to be included in COVID-19 vaccine trials. I spoke about the need to shift our mind-set from protecting pregnant women from being *included* in trials, to protecting them from being *excluded*.

I was shocked at how paternalistic viewer responses were, and at the overwhelming concern expressed for the fetus and unborn baby, but rarely any toward the pregnant woman.

I was also taken aback at how the general public still just assumes that women can't be trusted to make decisions about their own health and bodies. It appeared as though everyone had an opinion about what pregnant women should do but little desire to ask the women themselves.

We should all want to know more, not less, about the impact of this historic vaccine on half the world's population—women. That includes women who are pregnant, may be pregnant, or are pregnant and don't know it. A lack of data can never be helpful, especially in the face of COVID. It just leads to more uncertainty around pregnancy itself, and our one real shot at ending this pandemic, which is the vaccine.

Once again, we are seeing the male-dominated world of science and medicine leave women out and treat our health as an afterthought instead of a focus. We are watching in real time how, in America, a fetus is given more consideration than the life of an adult woman.

"As it turns out, pregnant women can be doctors and nurses and respiratory therapists," Dr. Emily Miller, assistant professor in the Division of Maternal-Fetal Medicine at Northwestern University's Feinberg School of Medicine, told the *Chicago Tribune*. She has been closely tracking the data on pregnant women and new vaccines, and agrees that it's putting our pregnant healthcare workers "in a place where they haven't been given a lot of concrete guidance because they've been systematically excluded."[32]

Experts are warning us to change course. The American College of Obstetricians and Gynecologists (ACOG) urged the CDC's Advisory Committee on Immunization Practices not to exclude women who are pregnant or lactating from the high-priority populations for COVID-19 vaccine allocation.[33] They pointed out that pregnant women are at high risk from the coronavirus in addition to being an at-risk group by themselves. More than half of pregnant women are also frontline workers *and* those with underlying conditions.[34]

What's even more outrageous is that pregnant women face the potential of severe illness from COVID, which can increase the risk of preterm birth and other serious health outcomes for both mother and infant.[35] Women twenty-eight weeks or more into a pregnancy are considered at increased risk if they contract the coronavirus, making it even more of a concern that they're not being included in trials.[36]

The sexist, incomplete, and lazy science of leaving pregnant women out of the trials is not only happening in America but also simultaneously around the world, as country after country rolls out a COVID vaccine. In Britain, regulators advised against offering the Pfizer-BioNTech vaccine to pregnant people or those who are breastfeeding, and also warned that "women of childbearing age should be advised to avoid pregnancy for at least 2 months after their second dose."[37] In Russia, the initial rollout of the Sputnik V vaccine did not include pregnant women, either.

While medical professionals are being vocal about pregnant women's higher risks, and they are speaking out about the negative aspects of excluding pregnant women, it is not changing the fact that for now, women are still left to make the decision whether to get vaccinated on their own.

"The precautionary principle when excluding pregnant and breastfeeding women from research doesn't ever think about how they might benefit from the research," Marian Knight, a professor of maternal and child population health at the University of Oxford, told the *Washington Post*.[38] She thinks the coronavirus pandemic offers a clear case for why this regulatory framework must change. "The default should be inclusion, unless there's a clear reason that women should be excluded."

So far, there is no red flag from either pharma company making the vaccine. Moderna released safety data on the vaccine in pregnant rats, finding "no vaccine-related adverse effects on female fertility, fetal development or postnatal development."[39] Neither did Pfizer's data from a similar study generate any big concerns for pregnant women.

This finding is consistent with past cases of pregnancy and vaccine. Except for the smallpox vaccine, which can cause a serious but rare fetal infection, vaccines have been generally safe and overwhelmingly beneficial for pregnant women and their babies. Experts say the new mRNA vaccines, which do not contain live virus, would probably be just as safe in both pregnant and nonpregnant people.[40]

Most experts also agree that the Pfizer and Moderna vaccines are unlikely to pose a risk to pregnant people, and ACOG is not giving preference for one vaccine over the other. The guidelines from the obstetricians and gynecologists group also conclude that in the absence of specific data, a pregnant woman should make an individual decision about whether to get vaccinated.[41]

Dr. Geeta Krishna Swamy is an ob-gyn at Duke University Medical Center who helped write the vaccine guidelines for the ACOG. She chose to be vaccinated and said early data from both vaccines reassured her that unless a woman is able to isolate at home during her pregnancy, the known risks of catching COVID-19 likely outweigh the theoretical risk of vaccination. Dr. Swamy said the vaccine has been shown to be safe and "is likely one of the most effective vaccines we've ever had."[42] The risk, according to her, "can never be zero without data," but so far there's nothing to suggest that pregnant women and their unborn children won't be safe.

"I personally feel comfortable recommending to those women that your risk-benefit balance suggests you should get vaccinated," Dr. Swamy said.[43] "If a woman says 'I don't want to get vaccinated,' I think that's absolutely, positively her choice, just like it's her choice to get vaccinated."

And for now, that's what women are doing—exercising their ability to choose. Maria Navarro, a frontline worker and an expectant mother, agrees with Dr. Swamy. Five months into her pregnancy with her first son, she did her research before receiving the vaccine.

"Seeing the science made me feel confident that the vaccine was going to be safe and effective—even in pregnancy," Navarro said.[44] "You want to do everything possible to defend and protect your kid? Then this is the single best way to fight against COVID. I encourage all moms to get vaccinated as well."

Ebony Marcelle is the director of midwifery at Community of Hope that includes Family Health and Birth Center. Formerly, as the administrative chief of midwifery service at MedStar Washington Hospital Center, she completed her nursing education at Georgetown University and midwifery at Philadelphia University. Ebony was recognized by the international organization Save the Children with their "Real Award Midwife Honoree" in 2014. She chose to get the COVID vaccine.

"As a midwife, I am a frontline worker, and we have seen many asymptomatic pregnant women finding out [they have COVID] with labor admission," Ebony said.[45] "I am also a mother to a nine-month-old who is nursing and [a] caretaker of [an] elderly parent. I can't afford, especially for them, to come home with COVID."

Ebony says aside from a sore arm and some fatigue, she was feeling normal the day after taking the vaccine but admits that being an African American woman was a big factor in her decision to get vaccinated.

"Yes, I was scared because I am a Black woman first before I am a provider," she says. "I carry generational distrust as well as my own history of trauma with medical systems. But understanding how the vaccine works and my potential risk of being exposed, I chose to do it . . . I'm hopeful that my daughter will also receive antibodies through my breast milk."

Other frontline women are additionally showing their confidence in the vaccine's safety and choosing to get vaccinated. Dr. Gayle Jordan, (not her real name), is a maternal-fetal medicine physician, and she says she is agonizing over getting the COVID vaccine.

"As a frontline healthcare worker, we are constantly in contact with patients who are COVID-19 positive," she said. "So the exposure risk and the infection risk for me is high."[46]

On top of working in a high-risk environment, Dr. Jordan is also pregnant. While the vaccine has been a welcome relief for her, Dr. Jordan says the lack of studies on pregnant women makes her anxiety worse.

"None of the clinical trials included pregnant or lactating women, so really we don't have the data for those groups," says Dr. Jordan. "I asked myself, 'If I don't get it now and then I get COVID-19, will I regret it?'"

Dr. Jordan decided to go for it, and at twenty-eight weeks, she got vaccinated. However, not all frontline workers are on the same page as Navarro, Marcelle, and Dr. Jordan. In online forums, some healthcare workers across the country expressed frustration over going first, with some saying it's a status associated with experimentation.

Glenda Ruiz, a medical center nurse, said healthcare workers wrestled with the same doubts, fears, and misinformation about the pandemic as the public. Though she interacts with other nurses who treat COVID patients, she's not getting the vaccine and knows others who aren't as well.

"I think the public perception of frontline workers is distorted," Ruiz said. "They might think we're all informed about COVID because we work in hospitals. But many people I work with are just as wary as the public. They are afraid of getting the vaccine, and I understand their apprehension."[47]

Melissa Lu is a thirty-one-year-old nurse who says she refused to get the vaccine because she is not convinced it is safe for pregnant women. At the time, Lu was six months pregnant. "I'm already risking COVID just by going to work," Lu said.[48] "But at least I have some degree of control by being careful, limiting my exposure, and wearing masks. I am aware it's not 100 percent going to keep me safe."

Lu said some of her coworkers also declined to get the vaccine because they've "made it this far" into the pandemic without getting the virus and also think they have a good shot at surviving it. "People think, 'I can take my chances, ride this out, and avoid risking the vaccine,'" Lu said.

The range of these women's stories shows how pregnant women are left on their own to make the agonizing decision of getting vaccinated against a raging pandemic—with no official guidelines. And experts' advice is not getting any clearer.

In late January 2021, major medical groups in the United States came out and told pregnant women to consider being vaccinated against COVID-19. "US regulatory bodies and medical experts have clearly stated that all eligible pregnant individuals should have the choice to receive the vaccine," said Dr. Christopher Zahn, vice president of practice activities for the American College of Obstetricians and Gynecologists.[49]

Dr. Richard Beigi, who sits on ACOG's Immunization, Infectious Disease, and Public Health Preparedness Expert Work Group, agrees with his colleague. "There's really no theoretical reason to believe it's going to cause harm to either the mother or her unborn child, and we're very confident it's going to provide considerable benefits to both the mother and the baby," he said in an interview to CNN.[50]

Both these statements came out the same week that the World Health Organization (WHO) recommended *against* getting the Moderna vaccine during pregnancy "unless the benefit of vaccinating a pregnant woman outweighs the potential vaccine risks."[51] The health agency also recommended against getting the Pfizer vaccine during pregnancy, pointing in both cases to a lack of safety data on pregnant women who were excluded from the original vaccine trial, stating that "due to insufficient data, WHO does not recommend the vaccination of pregnant women at this time," the Pfizer page states.[52]

So, basically, in the absence of any testing done on pregnant women and still no official guidelines, we are now telling pregnant women they should get vaccinated despite the CDC and the WHO essentially giving out conflicting advice?

In online pregnancy forums, women's views and concerns were all over the place, from not wanting to take the vaccine, which "may put my baby in danger," to responses from other women urging fellow expectant mothers to wait for more data, to healthcare workers saying they were "absolutely getting it."

Even for pregnant people who are able to stay healthy, carrying a child in a pandemic still brings a whole new level of worry and stress—especially for those at the lower end of the socioeconomic spectrum.

"Everywhere pregnant people turn, it's a little harder to make a decision," Dr. Marta Perez, an ob-gyn at Washington University School of Medicine in St. Louis, told *The Atlantic*.[53] "That can really wear on you."

Perez sees many women who are worried about losing their homes or jobs during the pandemic and who struggle to access healthcare. "This has been a year full of disappointment and hard decisions for families—not having family and friends around, not having child care—[and] making decisions brings an extra weight in terms of keeping yourself safe and boundaries for family members after the baby comes," she said. [54] "And now we have this decision about vaccine if it's offered to them."

Dr. Ruth Faden, a bioethicist at Johns Hopkins University who specializes in the health and rights of pregnant women, says successful inoculation against COVID means that pregnant and breastfeeding women must be included. She says that in clinical trials, a combination of ethical concerns and legal liability continues to handicap progress. "It's a profound injustice that pregnant women and offspring are late to the table and late to receive benefits," Faden said in an interview to the BBC.[55]

When we know better, we should do better, as the saying goes. But today, right before our eyes, during one of the most destructive pandemics in recent history, amid the creation of perhaps the most anticipated vaccine of our lifetimes, researchers are leaving out women. Again! It is outrageous and dangerous. Now is the time for women to demand that our health be prioritized—especially in a pandemic.

Even *The Lancet*, one of the most respected medical journals in the world, came out and said that despite the surge in treatment studies for COVID, the exclusion of pregnant women "remains consistent."[56] The journal said there was no good reason for excluding pregnant women from trials and called for pregnant women to be included so they could be effectively treated for COVID.

Why does such a simple suggestion sound so revolutionary? Women and experts continue to speak out in favor of pregnant women's inclusion in vaccine trials. So what are we waiting for? If

2020 taught us anything, it should be that we cannot afford to ignore women's health—and that we all pay when we do.

"We cannot have an effective vaccine against this pandemic unless we have a vaccine that pregnant women can take, full stop," Dr. Faden said to the BBC.[57]

Full stop, indeed. But what infuriates me even more about women being left out of such a critical clinical trial is that if there was ever a year when we saw what women were made of, especially moms, it was 2020. That was the year we saw how moms in America were hit by the pandemic—and how we were left with no choice but to tackle COVID head-on, with little or no help.

In the early days of the pandemic, even when we were told that lockdown would last initially for two weeks, I dreaded getting out of bed. While I suffered from low-grade depression and have been on a very "light" antidepressant since the birth of my first child, unlike most of my American friends, I was never in denial about what COVID presented—or how bad things could get. After all, I grew up in Bangladesh. I know what pandemics look like. I never imagined I would see one in the United States of America, but when COVID came, I recognized it immediately.

The lockdown had only just begun, but I knew nothing was going to be the same again. I had never seen the American people asked to give up anything for the "greater good," or for the larger health of our fellow citizens. I felt we were about to engage in war, not with a tangible enemy but with a virus. I had never seen Americans asked to sacrifice anything—even something as minor as forgoing restaurant dining.

But more than that, I was sad that the "protection" and security

I thought I had secured for my children was gone. COVID was the first time I truly felt unsafe in America. The pandemic shattered the lies I would tell myself about giving my kids a "first world" life despite having grown up in the "third world" myself, albeit extremely privileged.

From my point of view as a mother in America, things only got worse as the lockdown continued. In a matter of days, my three-year-old daughter couldn't go to the neighborhood park anymore. A few weeks in, my nanny left, over valid fears of infecting her family by helping me take care of mine.

Then, my elder daughter's elementary school shut down, like thousands of schools across the country. All of a sudden, I became a pseudo–fourth grade teacher and virtual-learning tech support for one kid, while providing full-time childcare for both kids. It was difficult, if not impossible, to continue my own work as a writer. Simultaneously, the main networks of support working women relied on began to disappear. Childcare and in-person schools in America suddenly didn't exist.

And I was one of the lucky women. I had a comfortable freelancing career, had been working from home way longer than most of my colleagues, and my husband is the primary breadwinner in our family. His tech company was able to survive the lethal impact the pandemic had on businesses everywhere, but there were definitely times we did not know if we would make it.

But as feminist and egalitarian as my marriage is, COVID nevertheless exposed traditional gender fault lines. As lockdown pushed everyone to start working from home, it also made the work of the person who made more money a priority. Before I knew it, my husband had taken over our home office, while I was relegated to the domestic sphere, as a reluctant 1950s-style housewife.

Initially, it was almost a foregone conclusion that my work should be set aside, at least temporarily. For a moment I saw my career disappearing before my eyes. Trapped at home: feeding, cleaning, educating, and entertaining my kids, I became a full-time mom. Every day, writing assignments and potential TV bookings slipped by.

Being responsible for providing my own childcare also meant I didn't really have the time to acknowledge or deal with depression. I was too busy and tired running after my kids during the day. I thought, "How did a privileged, highly educated Bangladeshi woman get trapped into the role of an American housewife? How did this happen to me?"

One day, I came across feminist author Helen Lewis's article in *The Atlantic* called "The Coronavirus Is a Disaster for Feminism."[58] The title alone terrified me, because I immediately knew she was right. The subtitle stated another truth: "Pandemics affect men and women differently."

"A pandemic magnifies all existing inequalities (even as politicians insist this is not the time to talk about anything other than the immediate crisis)," Lewis wrote. "But one of the most striking effects of the coronavirus will be to send many couples back to the 1950s. Across the world, women's independence will be a silent victim of the pandemic."[59]

Lewis said that it makes sense for many couples to make choices that make the most "economic sense,"[60] but points out that it will be women who will sacrifice more—especially career-wise.

"What do pandemic patients need?" Lewis asked. "Looking after. What do self-isolating older people need? Looking after. What do children kept home from school need? Looking after. All this looking after—this unpaid caring labor—will fall more heavily on women, because of the existing structure of the workforce."[61]

Lewis's words shook me to the core. Like so many women, I was already experiencing what she was predicting. So I went to my husband with an ultimatum: either we change the way we're splitting the day and our childcare responsibilities, or we get a divorce. It was quite a dramatic move, but I had to make clear that I couldn't continue with our initial pandemic setup.

Within twenty-four hours, we successfully negotiated "office hours." We agreed how we would share domestic labor and childcare. It made me realize that up until that point, as supportive as my husband had always been of my work, it was the nanny who was making it possible for me to pursue my writing career. For my husband, I was that support. The person who made his day run smoothly was me. In a COVID world, that had to change.

As helpful as it was to get time during the day carved out for my work and away from my kids, my depression lingered. I called my doctor to increase the low dosage of antidepressants he had put me on since the birth of my first daughter, almost a decade earlier, mostly as a precaution, since the condition runs rampant on my mother's side of the family.

Over the years, my antidepressants became an emotional and chemical crutch that I relied on to keep more serious depression at bay. In a COVID world, I needed that support more than ever, this time not only to get me out of bed but also to help me muster enough energy to be emotionally present for my kids.

This is how trapped and hopeless I was feeling despite all the privileges afforded by my upper northwest Washington, DC, neighborhood; despite having good health insurance and being able to call a doctor and get a prescription to treat my mental health. This is how alone I felt inside, despite the neighborhood moms coming together to set up learning "pods" for our kids. Some of us hired tutors and took turns hosting a "lunch bunch" so our children could get a break from their computer screens in order to enjoy some human interaction with their friends. We also checked in on one another by having our "pandemic mom happy hours" regularly.

Yet, my mental health was still steadily falling apart. If I felt I were drowning despite staying afloat, what the hell were other women across America feeling? The answer, in neon lights, is DE-PRESSED. Depression is number one on the list of the most urgent women's health issues.

Is this really a surprise? It is not an overstatement to say American women's lives unraveled during COVID. Women are bearing the brunt of the pandemic, and we have the numbers to prove it. With no other social safety nets in place, the gendered impact of COVID was obvious from the start, and women started paying the price from the get-go.

By the fall of 2020, 865,000 women had left the US workforce, four times more than men.[62] Women of color, particularly Latina women, were hit hardest—nearly three times more than white women, and four times more than Black women.[63] In December 2020, women accounted for *all* 140,000 of US job losses, clearly reflecting the pandemic's disastrous impact on working women, especially women of color.[64]

Things are unlikely to get better for women anytime soon. Journalist and author Hanna Rosin wrote in a recent article for *New York* magazine, "The End of the End of Men,"[65] that women had everything stacked against us from when we started entering the workforce.

It's now painfully obvious that the mass entry of women into the workforce was rigged from the beginning. American work culture has always conspired to keep professional women out and working-class women shackled. Add to that late capitalism's stagnant wages, making it nearly impossible to support a family on one salary. As with so many things, the pandemic just exposed what should have been obvious all along.[66]

Rosin points to the timing of 865,000 women dropping out of the workforce in the fall of 2020 compared with 216,000 men during the same period. "What complex confluence of demographic shifts converged at that critical time?" Rosin asked.[67] The answer, of course, is the start of school.

"Parents of little kids had already experimented in the previous school year with trying to do their own work while serving as teachers' assistants and realized it was impossible," Rosin wrote. "When September came around, they wisely opted for just one of those jobs."[68]

Rosin is clear about who she is talking about when she says "they"—women. She cites research done by Misty Heggeness, a research economist at the US Census Bureau, who has been tracking young families on a weekly basis, state by state, and finds that the "impact on short-term work productivity and engagement appeared to be borne entirely on the backs of mothers of school-age children."[69]

Rosin urges her readers to look for "humanity and pathos"[70] behind those numbers because they represent real women's struggles. Her article warns that the hard work and progress toward closing the gender wage gap could be set back decades. But she says it's more about the work interruption than wages.

Rosin points to a study that found that women who took just one year out of the workforce had annual earnings that were 39 percent lower than those of women who didn't. That number is worse for Black women, who have higher rates of work participation than white women, but also much higher rates of work disruptions. "It's like working in quicksand," Rosin wrote. "You will never, ever, be able to get ahead."[71]

It is not just that more women are losing, or voluntarily leaving, their jobs. They are also more exhausted from the combined demands of childcare and housework. That women report higher levels of depression than men is nothing new. The pandemic is increasing these feelings among women with children as they are forced to work, parent, and teach—simultaneously and with little or no support.

With nationwide school closures, there were 1.6 million fewer mothers in the labor force in 2020.[72] According to the Census Bureau, a third of working women twenty-five to forty-four years old who are currently unemployed pointed to lack of available childcare as the reason, versus only 12 percent of unemployed men.[73] A 2020 paper out of the University of Southern California found that in two-adult, mixed-gender households it's generally women who were more likely to report psychological distress following the pandemic—especially for women with children.[74]

"My spouse is a physician in the emergency dept, and is actively treating #coronavirus patients," Emory University epidemiologist Rachel Patzer, mother to a newborn and two young children, wrote in a viral thread of tweets in March 2020. "We just made the difficult decision for him to isolate & move into our garage apartment for the foreseeable future as he continues to treat patients. . . . As I attempt to homeschool my kids (alone) with a new baby who screams if she isn't held, I am worried about the health of my spouse and my family."[75]

Should it surprise us, then, that 74 percent of American moms say they feel mentally worse since the pandemic began? A 2020 *Motherly* report, an online platform to support mothers, surveyed more than three thousand moms between March 9 and April 23 in their annual "State of Motherhood" report. They found that 97 percent of moms between the ages of twenty-four and thirty-nine agreed that the pandemic was making their burnout worse, with 30 percent of full-time working moms saying that their primary cause of stress is childcare.[76]

COVID is also dramatically affecting the mental health of pregnant women. "Women are expressing so much fear about being infected, but also about going to the hospital, delivering and being separated from their child," Laura Jelliffe-Pawlowski told the *New York Times*.[77] She is an epidemiologist who is the primary investigator of HOPE COVID-19, a new study that investigates how COVID-19 and the pandemic response impacts pregnancy. Her team is finding "absolutely incredible"[78] levels of stress and anxiety in women.

"Sixty percent of women are experiencing nervousness and anxiety at levels that impede their everyday functioning," Dr. Jelliffe-Pawlowski told the *Times*. "There are a number of women, particularly lower-income women, expressing how hard it is to choose to stay in a job that puts them at risk versus quitting the job and not having enough food for their baby."[79]

Dr. Jelliffe-Pawlowski said she doubts women are getting the psychological care they need. "If you can't feed your family, seeking out mental health care is not your top priority."[80]

Another 2020 study published in the online publication for maternal health *Frontiers in Global Women's Health* found the pandemic is exacerbating struggles with anxiety and depression during the perinatal period. The platform's study, titled "Moms Are Not

OK," surveyed nine hundred women (520 were pregnant and 380 had given birth in the past year) and found that the likelihood of maternal depression and anxiety has substantially increased during this health crisis.[81]

Prior to the pandemic, 29 percent of those women surveyed experienced moderate to high anxiety symptoms, and 15 percent experienced depressive symptoms. But during COVID, those numbers almost tripled: 72 percent of women said they experienced anxiety, and 41 percent said they experienced depression.[82]

Lynda Hernandez says her newborn son keeps her busy. "I went to work five weeks after he was born," Hernandez, the owner of a small physical fitness business, said.[83] The first-time mom said having a baby in the middle of a pandemic no doubt made her anxious, stressed, and depressed.

"The most difficult part was not being able to share the birth of my child with family, and not being able to rely on them for what a new mom needs as well," she recalled. Hernandez said it was only a matter of time before the postpartum isolation due to COVID brought on feelings of postpartum depression. "Feeling a sense of such loss at the same time as welcoming your newborn baby . . . I just really was not understanding what was going on with my body or my mind. And I was all alone."

Single parent Corrine Hudson says the pandemic was not at the forefront of her mind when she went into labor in the spring of 2020. She had a complicated birth that ended in an emergency C-section. Hudson even says that giving birth in a pandemic had its "perks."[84]

"It was kind of nice, and I felt relieved not to have to put on a brave face to visitors," she said. "My baby and I spent the first couple of weeks at home, working out what we were doing. Our antenatal classes had all been online, but we'd all been shown how to do the basics, like putting a diaper on. I had also reached out to some neighborhood moms to meet up as soon as lockdown was lifted."[85]

But what Hudson didn't anticipate was having trouble breast-feeding. She said she found herself in tears not only because the baby wasn't feeding but because it was so frustrating that no one could come to her house to help her. No lactation consultant, friend, or another fellow new mom. Hudson's own mother does not live close by. "I just needed someone to tell me if I was doing it right, if the baby was normal," Hudson said. "I was terrified my baby was starving."[86]

Six weeks into being a new mom, struggling to breastfeed her baby in the isolation of lockdown, Hudson said she started to scream. "I felt so alone in terms of medical support," Hudson recalled. "It was only when I spoke to friends with similar-aged babies that I realized it wasn't normal. Eventually, I found a doctor to see in person, who diagnosed my baby with acid reflux."[87]

Hudson says she was lucky to be able to afford an out-of-network private doctor, but she worries about other women who are struggling. "There must be so many new mothers who are struggling," she said. "Think about all the women's stories we don't know. They are falling through the cracks."[88]

Pregnant women and new mothers must also deal with the "constant low-grade panic"[89] that comes with making decisions that have no specific medical guidelines, such as: What should I do if I have other kids at home and the only person who can help me is a grandparent who is at high risk? What kind of precautions should I take if my partner is a healthcare worker? Is it OK to send my kid back to school? Without clear guidance from the government or the CDC, the mental load of these decisions falls on women who are already stretched to their limits.

Ines Moina, thirty-six, feels that everything is coming together for her in a perfect storm. She's just waiting for it to crash. Moina, a government contractor, said her mental health worsened with the pandemic. On some days, she can barely get out of bed. Moina works from home with her two children. Since separating from her husband, she is now the primary caretaker and homeschooler in her family.

The burden is overwhelming, Moina said, especially when it comes to dealing with virtual learning for her children. Her eleven-year-old daughter Zooms her way through a sixth-grade school day in what used to be Moina's home office. But Moina's seven-year-old sits with her at the dining room table, which is "covered with colored folders, workbooks, markers, crayons, and pencils."[90] While she tries to focus on the silver lining of being home with her kids, Moina is aware that if both her kids don't go back to in-person learning soon, she will have no option but to quit her job.

"I live in my children's school," Moina told me. "I'm sitting right there, listening along, helping find the right workbook, making sure they're eating. I am so stressed out that I can't work on most days. Their school time was my work time. When do I get that back?"

Moina is already seeing the psychological burden affect other aspects of her health. Painful and "physically draining" migraines are becoming more and more frequent.

"I pray my health doesn't worsen and that I [don't] have to be hospitalized," she said. "This is not the time to go to the hospital. I could get COVID just by going to the ER."

Like Moina, Nadiya Hussein finds there is no one to support her as she tries to keep her family healthy, educated, and fed. Throughout her years as a working mother climbing the corporate ladder, Hussein tried to be home for dinner with her kids. Now, the pandemic has kept her home full-time.

"I respect stay-at-home moms, but it's not something I ever wished for," said Hussein, who spent almost two decades climbing the corporate ladder.[91] "I loved the hustle and bustle of my work. I loved being good at my job."

With COVID, work became so stressful that Hussein, an assistant vice president at a public relations company, had to lay people off. At home, her family life was also facing emotional challenges. Hussein's husband works as a truck driver and stayed away from home for a month out of fear of passing the virus on to his family. Hussein had no option but to leave her job.

"My family needs me," Hussein told me, trying not to cry. "It was a tough decision, but what is the alternative? I had to stay home with my kids because that is exactly where they need me to be."

That is precisely the message the pandemic is sending to a lot of women: home is where you need to be. Kimberly Shaffer, thirty-eight, is mom to three teenagers. She said figuring out homeschooling has been the biggest source of stress and anxiety for her—even bigger than her financial worries. Shaffer can't rely on family because her job as an essential worker puts her at risk. She also worries about which of her kids she should send back to in-person school.

"Putting one of my kids back on campus could put my other kids at risk," Shaffer said.[92] She also admits that dealing with the stress of being your child's educator is one of the biggest challenges she has ever dealt with.

Even women with high-profile, well-paying jobs are suffering. Tanzina Vega is a journalist who reported for the *New York Times* and CNN. She is currently the host of *The Takeaway*, a public radio show broadcast on hundreds of radio stations. In January 2021, she sent out a tweet about something many have called the "pandemic wall."[93] The tweet went viral in a few hours and was shared everywhere, from Hawaii to Spain.

"Lots of people—including me—are hitting what I'm calling the pandemic wall this week," Vega tweeted. "The burnout from working non stop, no break from news, childcare and isolation is hard. It's ok not to be ok right now. I think we need to accept that."[94]

This is not how it should be for women in America. When you look at how women across the board are faring in the richest country in the world, with everything asked of us in the absence of modest amounts of childcare, it is shocking that more mothers are not screaming from the rooftops. COVID may have revealed the holes in America's healthcare system, but more significantly, it has exposed the tremendous pressure society piles on women.

"Other countries have social safety nets; the US has women," Jessica Calarco, a sociologist at Indiana University, told journalist Anne Helen Petersen in an interview for her newsletter, *Culture Study*.[95] "Women in the US have long done a disproportionate share of the unpaid service work in institutions and at home. They're the ones who run the bake sales so the school can have an art teacher or enough books to go around. They're the ones who run church outreach programs to attract new families and serve community members in need. They're the ones who check in on sick coworkers, remember birthdays, and help their colleagues feel like part of a team. Women do all of that unpaid service for the institutions in their lives, and then they go home and do even more."[96]

Calarco tells Petersen in their interview that American women serve as the social safety net because norms that serve capitalistic, patriarchal, and white interests tell them that's their role. She says breaking those norms leaves them open to judgments, or worse, from others, not to mention their own self-imposed guilt trips.[97]

"The pandemic came along and ripped a giant hole through what little safety net we did have to support women and especially mothers in the US," Calarco said. "It's closed the childcare centers and schools mothers rely on for childcare; it's made it more difficult for mothers to rely on other people and organizations they might usually turn to for support. And because of the pandemic's disproportionate impact on women's careers, it has also made it more difficult for unpartnered mothers to support their families and for mothers in difficult or dangerous relationships to consider leaving and going out on their own."[98]

Calarco warns that we are not paying enough attention to how mothers are struggling to stay in the workforce while caring for their children at home. These women could face penalties like being passed over for promotions or salary increases, or being chastised by their bosses for failing to get work done on time. "But these women are also taking serious hits to their relationships, their health, and their wellbeing."[99]

The pandemic also exposed how the many burdens of the pandemic-induced recession fell most heavily on low-income and minority women and single mothers.

"When the pandemic hit, it was largely mothers who took on the additional child care duties; became remote teachers; and, in large numbers, quit their jobs," Pulitzer Prize–winning *New York Times* correspondent Claire Cain Miller wrote. "The sudden return to 1950s-style households wasn't an aberration. Rather, it revealed a truth: In the United States, mothers remain the fallback plan."[100]

And it does not look as if the load is going to lighten any time soon. With vaccine rollout underway in America, feminist author Jessica Valenti predicts that women will bear the burden of getting our aging parents vaccinated, just as we have been doing the bulk of childcare.

"American women, who overwhelmingly are tasked with caretaking for senior parents, now have another huge responsibility added to their already very full plate of child rearing and domestic work,"[101] Valenti wrote. "The pandemic over the past year has hit women in this country particularly hard: Women are losing their jobs at a much higher rate than their male counterparts . . . It's a gap that experts predict could undo decades of economic progress. All because of the expectation that women should be the ones primarily responsible for care work—not just childcare, but eldercare as well."

Valenti warns that while it's easy to lose sight of just how thinly stretched half the country's population is, if we don't start to pay attention to the outsized burden on American women, employment and domestic work disparities that already feel untenable will turn into a full-on disaster.[102]

None of this bodes well for women's mental health, the complications of which are further compounded by race. While people of color experienced more mental health issues even before the pandemic, the stresses associated with the pandemic have made those disparities even worse.

Since the end of April 2020, Black and Latina women were more likely than white women to report depression or anxiety, though the gap has fluctuated over the course of the pandemic, according to data from the CDC.[103] At the end of June 2020, 47.9 percent of Latina women and 45.8 percent of Black women reported symptoms of at least one condition, compared to 38.7 percent of white women.[104]

Black women, in particular, are dealing with an acute mental health challenge that other groups of women aren't. On top of the pandemic, the nationwide upheaval over police brutality has understandably taken a serious psychological toll on the mental health of Black women.

The Black Lives Matter (BLM) movement brought an international spotlight on racism in America. The stories of Black women like Breonna Taylor, who was asleep in her bed, and Atatiana Jefferson, who was playing video games with her nephew, being shot by the police in their own homes added to the already heavy emotional load Black women carry.

In fact, the CDC's mental health figures showed a significant increase in Black women's rates of depression and anxiety starting on May 26, 2020, the day after George Floyd's death at the hands of the police. That spike didn't appear for any other group of women—white, Asian, or Latina.[105]

"We and our colleagues are well versed in diagnosing depression and anxiety," Brandi Jackson, a cofounding director of the Institute for Antiracism in Medicine and an adjunct professor of psychiatry at Rush University Medical Center, wrote in the *Washington Post*.[106] "Some of us suffer from it ourselves. But what all Black women are facing today is something different, something additional. Black women sit squarely at the confluence of multiple systems of oppression, and are experiencing a disproportionate loss of life and livelihood in the era of COVID-19."

Jackson says that researchers are only just beginning to understand the extent of racism's impact on mental health, which she described as a "powerful layer on top of the stressors imposed by COVID-19 and its economic fallout."[107]

"The impact of discrimination and living in fear on Black women's mental health cannot be overstated and is a huge source of anxiety and stress," wrote Lynya Floyd, former health director at *Family Circle*. "Black women see a constant barrage of news and videos of people who look like them and those they love being killed driving while Black, jogging while Black, or sleeping while Black. We feel for our friends and family who are experiencing racial trauma, even if we are not directly affected."[108]

The lack of research into Black people's specific mental health concerns is also a big problem because it leads to a lack of information on what works for the community. A study from 2000 even found that African Americans seeking treatment for mental health issues are less likely to be offered evidence-based medication, therapy, or psychotherapy.[109]

Dr. Sirry Alang, chair of the Health Justice Collaborative at Lehigh University and author of a recent study on mental health among Black people, tells *Prevention* magazine that most of what we know about "evidence-based"[110] treatments has been developed by research and experiments done on white people, and so it isn't necessarily applicable to African Americans.

"With the dual pandemics of racism and COVID-19 upon us, Black women are overwhelmed," Dr. Angela Neal-Barnett, a professor of psychological sciences and the director of the Program for Research on Anxiety Disorders Among African Americans at Kent State University, told *Prevention*.[111] "We don't have time to explain to a therapist what it means to be Black and female in this country. We don't have the energy to educate our therapists about who we are as Black women."

Sherri Williams, an assistant professor at American University's School of Communication, writes that as a Black woman, she felt the need to keep her mental health struggles to herself. Williams says that depression has been a constant part of her life since she was eight years old.[112]

"Like most Black people, it's not something I talk about openly with everyone," Williams wrote in *Self*. "I'm already Black, a woman, and overweight. Why add another stigmatized identity? Why give people another reason to doubt my capability? Why threaten my professional reputation? Why be vulnerable? As a community, some of us either suffer in silence or keep our mental health issues between us and the Lord."[113]

However, Williams also recognizes that that silence is killing her community. With the racial justice protests that erupted across the country over the summer of 2020, she says it is imperative to study, talk about, and remove the stigma around race and mental health.

Let us look at the case of Ferguson, Missouri. In the days after the 2014 shooting of Michael Brown, an unarmed Black teenager, by a white police officer, the St. Louis suburb erupted in protests. As demonstrators and police clashed, military tanks drove down neighborhood streets. St. Louis clinical psychologist Marva Robinson, PsyD, told *Self* magazine that she witnessed her community "traumatized, devastated, torn apart, and left without the appropriate resources to help it rebuild."[114]

A 2016 study published in the *Journal of Traumatic Stress* also found that Black residents of Ferguson had significantly higher rates of post-traumatic stress disorder and depression than white residents in the months following the protests.[115] Williams says that the tragedy in Ferguson, and the psychological toll it took on people there, was at once an extreme example and a microcosm of the damaging effects of institutionalized racism in this country.

But there is also a racial and cultural gap when it comes to seeking and accepting treatment for mental health in communities of color. According to federal data, Black and Latina women are particularly vulnerable to symptoms of anxiety and depression but are also less likely than their white counterparts to seek treatment.[116]

"The root structure of psychology, and much of what's been baked into even the foundations of mental health, has been stigmatizing and not at all supportive in meeting the needs of communities of color," Dr. Joy Harden Bradford, a clinical psychologist who started the blog *Therapy for Black Girls*, told ABC News. She points out that therapy is "just a very foreign concept" to women of color, and her goal is to create space for Black women to talk about their mental health.[117]

Williams echoes this in her writing and talks about struggling to be open about her own struggles because of the "strong Black woman" stereotype.

"For years people told me they saw me as a strong Black woman," Williams wrote in *Self*. "I always hated being associated with the strong Black woman archetype because it's an unhealthy and unrealistic myth that forces black women to carry the world on our backs while crumbling inside and not being allowed to talk about it. Yet at the same time, I hesitated to include my depression in the story because I didn't want to be perceived as weak. I know that experiencing depression or any kind of mental distress isn't weak, it's part of being human. But we live in a society that doesn't allow Black people to be human, vulnerable or have emotions."[118]

Williams recognizes that's exactly why writing her own story is important, because "acknowledging the range of feelings that black people experience also recognizes our humanity and resists ideas about us being devoid of emotions."[119]

Williams is far from alone. Experts find that women from

communities of color often try to manage depression and anxiety on their own—a habit that can prove to be especially harmful during a pandemic of COVID's proportion.

"You're not supposed to tell strangers your secrets," Alysha Pamphile, a thirty-four-year-old Haitian American living in New Jersey, told ABC News. "There's such a taboo around therapy, and the space of being vulnerable, a sense of weakness, when in fact, it's quite the opposite. But we weren't given the language to do that; we hadn't been allowed that grace."[120]

Zahra Haider's story reflects exactly that lack of "grace." She was a nineteen-year-old student when she first considered suicide before opting for therapy. But it wasn't easy. Haider didn't have any friends or family who had seen a therapist before, so her search was self-directed and self-motivated. On top of that, she faced growing stigma from her Pakistani American community.

"For Black and Brown people know, feeling shame around mental illness is something that is passed down through the generations—especially around depression," she said.[121] "African American, Latino, and Desi cultures think depression and other mental illnesses are meant to be prayed away, ignored." Haider says that many of these cultures encourage keeping mental health problems to yourself.

According to the Centers for Medicare and Medicaid Services Office of Minority Health report, depression is the most common mental health condition across all minorities. Puerto Ricans have the highest rate of depression at 40 percent, Black people at 27 percent, and American Indian and Alaskan Native Americans at 9 percent above white Medicare beneficiaries.[122] And these statistics are from 2019, so the situation was already in dire straits before the pandemic.

In the era of COVID, not only is depression spiking for women and communities of color, but the same barriers that are disproportionately affecting their mental health—e.g., childcare, extra housework, and financial worries—also make it harder to put aside money for mental health treatment or therapy. According to a 2020 Pew Research survey, an additional barrier for women of color is that many are from "collectivistic cultures,"[123] which emphasize the needs and goals of the group as a whole over the needs and desires of individuals.

Pew's data found that 29 percent of Asian Americans, 27 percent of Hispanics, and 26 percent of African Americans live in multigenerational family households.[124] Women of color have to think not only of themselves but also their extended family members *and* wider communities.

For women of color, the biggest health concern is not just how to manage depression in the COVID era, but how to survive the pandemic itself. Even before the pandemic, women of color stood at the intersection of gender, race, and class. The pandemic has taken the lid off this reality for all to see. The *New York Times* said this pandemic has a predominantly nonwhite, female face.[125] But what does that actually mean?

From healthcare to home care, restaurants to grocery stores, women, specifically women of color, are on the front lines of the COVID-19 pandemic. Nearly 80 percent of healthcare workers and 83 percent of workers who provide social assistance, including childcare and emergency services, are women.[126] After depression, COVID is the second biggest women's health issue in America today.

We can see how the intersection of race and gender are compounded for communities of color when we examine the immense toll the pandemic has taken on New York's Filipino American community, a crucial part of the fabric of hospitals in New York City. The investigative journalism nonprofit ProPublica reports that Filipinos are four times more likely to be nurses than any other ethnic group in the United States, and in the New York–New Jersey region, nearly a quarter of adults with Filipino ancestry work in hospitals or other medical fields.[127]

Many also live in Elmhurst and Woodside in Queens—a.k.a. Little Manila—neighborhoods that were among the hardest hit during COVID. According to a September 2020 study by National Nurses United, the largest nurses' union in the United States, almost a third of all the nurses who died from the pandemic nationwide were Filipino.[128]

Belinda Ellis was a nurse for forty years working in hospitals in the Philippines, Saudi Arabia, and even a military hospital on the border of Iraq. Ellis, now sixty-five, says she is still "shaken"[129] by the memory of New York's Elmhurst Hospital in March and April 2020. She was assigned to the hospital's COVID-19 unit. "I've worked in Iraq at the height of a war," she said in an interview to the *New York Times*. "This was worse."[130]

According to the *Times*, Filipinos are overrepresented in the types of healthcare professions that require close contact with patients, such as in emergency rooms and nursing homes. This is a risk increased by the high numbers of hypertension, asthma, obesity, and diabetes among Filipinos.[131]

"Everything has been pointing to the risk for Filipino healthcare workers," Ninez Ponce, a researcher at UCLA's Fielding School of Public Health who studies health disparities, told the *Times*.[132]

Kevin Nadal is a professor of psychology at John Jay College of Criminal Justice and the Graduate Center of the City University of New York who has written extensively about Filipino American psychology and culture. He says the scale of the trauma and the way it is unfolding are "similar to times of war."[133]

The combat metaphor is echoed by Laarni Florencio, a board member of the Philippine Nurses Association of New York. She said in an interview to the *Times* that in the spring of 2020, when the pandemic was ravaging New York, many Filipino nurses went weeks without sleeping at home. She began providing mental health Zoom calls for the group's members.[134]

"Our hospitals look like battlegrounds," she said. "We were hearing stories about how depressed the nurses feel, about how they were crying at work. That emotional toll for health care providers is tough. We're supposed to be healers."[135]

According to a survey published in September by National Nurses United, 67 Filipino nurses have died of COVID-19. That number is about a third of the total registered nurses who have died nationwide, though Filipinos make up only 4 percent of registered nurses overall.[136]

"It's really heartbreaking," Zenei Cortez, president of National Nurses United and a nurse from the Philippines herself, said. She fears that the true statistics are worse. "The numbers we are producing are all underreported, I'm sure of that."[137]

Fordham University law professor Catherine Powell says for women of color, the COVID pandemic exposes all the race-based inequalities they live with—from jobs to healthcare to the "broader racial justice paradoxes" of American life. Powell writes that people of color are more likely to be unemployed yet also more likely to be those essential workers who must stay on their jobs, particularly lower-skill jobs, such as those at Amazon fulfillment centers.[138]

While women of color dominate in domestic work, they have zero job security, and many are not working due to the pandemic.

Powell's work also highlights who has the *privilege* of working from home. Again, racial and class inequities are a major factor. According to the Bureau of Labor Statistics, while 37 percent of Asian workers and 29.9 percent of white workers are able to work remotely, only 19.7 percent of Black workers and 16.2 percent of Latino workers are able to do so.[139] These are the people who have no choice but to leave their homes and show up for work during a pandemic.

"While millions of white-collar employees now work remotely from home, jobless claims have once again soared . . . with people of color particularly hard hit," Powell wrote in an op-ed for CNN. "Meanwhile, 'essential' workers largely can't work from home. They include not only doctors and other frontline health workers, but also blue-collar workers, such as grocery cashiers, delivery workers, bus drivers, mail carriers and warehouse workers."[140]

Given this reality, Powell says that COVID has "forever colored"[141] our understanding of not only the crisis of contagion but also the ethics of community, care, and concern. She states that we must all reconcile—and address—the fact that Black and Latino communities and women are bearing the brunt of the pandemic.[142]

In addition to depression, and the pandemic itself, COVID is also wreaking havoc on women's sexual and reproductive health. While I discuss the pandemic, pregnancy, and maternal health in depth in the next chapter, it is important to mention here yet another gendered aspect of COVID—making women across the country delay pregnancy.

A 2020 report from the reproductive health research organization the Guttmacher Institute found that, unsurprisingly, COVID is making women put off pregnancy. Guttmacher surveyed 2,009 women and found that one-third of women say they now want to delay having children or want fewer children. The same number of women also said the pandemic made them change their attitude toward contraception with one-third indicating that they are now "more careful" than before about using birth control.[143]

A 2020 report from the Brookings Institution estimated that the United States would see as many as 500,000 fewer births in 2021, a 13 percent drop from the 3.8 million babies born in 2019.[144] The telehealth clinic Nurx told *Time* it has seen a 50 percent increase in requests for birth control since the beginning of the pandemic and a 40 percent increase in requests for the emergency contraception pill, Plan B.[145]

A survey from the Guttmacher also found that 34 percent of sexually active women in the United States have decided to either delay getting pregnant or have fewer children because of concerns arising from COVID. Not surprisingly, lower-income women were much more likely than other women to want to put off having a baby, especially Black and Latina women, who have been hit harder with loss of income and jobs.[146]

The long-term impact of women delaying pregnancy has serious implications for the American economy. The US fertility rate is the lowest it has been since 1985, and as a relatively elderly nation, we are also facing a serious shortage of workers and people to care for an aging population.[147]

Women's rights advocates point out that the "looming baby bust"[148] says a lot about quality, or lack thereof, of healthcare and childcare systems in the United States. Let's not forget that America is the only developed country that does not guarantee paid family leave, and it does not offer universal childcare or universal pre-K. The pandemic has made every aspect of being a mother harder—

and likely has not inspired a lot of confidence in women contemplating motherhood.

"COVID set off a bomb in the middle of these jerry-rigged ways of getting by in this country that individual families had created," Emily Martin of the National Women's Law Center told *Time*. "It's no wonder parents don't want to deal with having a newborn right now."[149]

Simultaneously, COVID is making it more challenging than ever for women to access birth control. One in three women surveyed said the pandemic made it harder for them to obtain birth control or has delayed or forced cancellations of their doctor visits.

Women of color are disproportionately affected by this, because Black and Hispanic women face bigger challenges getting care than white women. The Guttmacher report found that 38 percent of Black women and 45 percent of Hispanic women reported issues with access to care, compared to just 29 percent of white women. There were also similar discrepancies for other marginalized groups like queer women (46 percent) when compared to straight women (31 percent).[150]

But while COVID has brought mayhem upon so many aspects of women's health that we can see, measure, and analyze, such as job numbers and mental health statistics, there is also a more invisible women's health crisis that the pandemic has exacerbated—domestic violence. After depression and COVID itself, this is the third biggest health issue facing American women today.

According to statistics from the National Coalition Against Domestic Violence, more than ten million women and men in the country survive domestic violence on a daily basis. The numbers were already stressful pre-COVID, especially for women of color.[151]

According to a 2018 report from the Department of Justice, 41 to 60 percent of Asian and Pacific Islander women have reported abuse; 37.5 percent and 23.4 percent of Native American and Latina women, respectively, said they were victimized by a partner at some point in their lives. Black women experience domestic violence 35 percent more than white women and two and a half times the rate of other women of color.[152]

The liberal policy think tank the Center for American Progress reports that domestic violence has surged as America continues to grapple with the devastation unleashed upon the country by COVID. Quarantine and stay-at-home orders essential to slowing the spread of the virus, on top of the economic and health stressors caused by the pandemic, forced survivors already at risk of domestic abuse into even more dangerous situations. For women across the country, the pandemic has created a double threat—the risk of getting COVID and the danger of being in lockdown with their abusers.[153]

"The first thing that came to mind when I heard about COVID restrictions and mitigation strategies was how exceptionally dangerous this time could be for women living with abusive partners," wrote Dr. Eve Valera, an assistant professor in psychiatry at Harvard Medical School and a research scientist at Massachusetts General Hospital. "Self-isolate," "stay at home," "practice social distancing," and "recession" are phrases likely to terrify many women who are living with intimate partner violence (IPV). The lives of these women are often filled with fear and danger under normal circumstances, but during this new normal of the global pandemic, the lives of these very often "invisible victims" are at an increased risk for more violence—and murder.[154]

Dr. Valera says that even before the COVID pandemic, epidemiological estimates showed that nearly one in three women experience IPV, and approximately one in four women experience *severe* IPV. Other data show that nearly half of all female homicides are from a current or past male intimate partner.[155]

Laila Qureshi's boyfriend had never been violent toward her, but she says everything changed when the first lockdown was put in place. "My boyfriend's existing mental health issues only got worse in lockdown," she recalled. She said that while she was already working from home and used to it, the pandemic restrictions made her boyfriend's anger issues come to a head.[156]

"He would get so angry out of nowhere, completely unprovoked," Qureshi recollects. She said he became unpredictable, and she suffered a series of physical attacks.[157]

One day, as Qureshi was in the shower, her boyfriend barged in on her and ripped open the shower curtain. "He pushed my face against the wall and started spitting on me and choking me," she told me. "Then he held me under the shower, under the hot water. It was boiling. I thought he was going to kill me."[158]

After months of attacks, Qureshi's boyfriend kicked her out, and she found herself homeless on her birthday. "I was terrified and had nowhere to go," she said. "But I was alive."

Tanisha Leaf said that when her boyfriend strangled her, she nearly died. "I woke up, I just felt numb," she recalled. "My whole body was just like, 'Am I here? Am I dead?'"[159]

Leaf says things escalated between her and her partner when she refused to cook him dinner. He put his hands around her neck and started to squeeze, strangling her in front of her children.

When Leaf's seven-year-old daughter tried to stop the assault on her mother "with her tiny balled-up fists," he paused just long enough to drag Leaf by her hair into another room, where he continued to strangle her and put a pillow over her face. Leaf lost consciousness. "He's strangled me before, but not to where I blacked out," she said. "I woke up and just like in a daze, and I was like, 'I have to get out of this house. I have to leave.'"

This happened in late April 2020. The whole state of Texas was locked down because of the coronavirus, and Leaf was faced with the same choices domestic abuse victims have been grappling with since the start of the pandemic: either to flee from abuse and violence or stay home to avoid COVID.

"I had to make a decision," Leaf said. "Should I leave right now during this pandemic and we could possibly get sick, or I need to go and save my life and my kids."

Although it's still early, studies and statistics are already showing a clear connection between the pandemic and surging domestic violence. An October 2020 article published in the *American Journal of Emergency Medicine* titled "Alarming Trends in US Domestic Violence During the COVID-19 Pandemic" warns that stay-at-home orders could cause a "catastrophic milieu"[160] for individuals whose lives are plagued by domestic violence.

The article also shows an alarming rise in domestic violence reported by police departments. In four cities across the country, the percent increase in domestic violence in 2020 is dramatic: 27 percent in Jefferson, Alabama; 22 percent in Portland, Oregon; 18 percent in San Antonio, Texas; and 10 percent in New York, New York.[161]

The economic stress and unemployment brought on by the pandemic-led recession only makes domestic violence worse. Due to the pandemic, US unemployment and overall financial stress are at an all-time high. Experts identify economic instability as a major risk factor for domestic violence, and find domestic violence more common in households experiencing financial stress or unemployment. There is also evidence suggesting that domestic violence increases in times of national crisis.[162]

The National Domestic Violence Hotline reports that a growing number of women are saying that their abusers are using the pandemic as a means of further isolating them from friends and family. "Perpetrators are threatening to throw their victims out on the street so they get sick," Katie Ray-Jones, the CEO of the National Domestic Violence Hotline, told *Time*. "We've heard of some withholding financial resources or medical assistance."[163]

"My husband won't let me leave the house," one victim of domestic violence told a representative for the National Domestic Violence Hotline over the phone, according to *Time*. "He's had flu-like symptoms, and blames keeping me here on not wanting to infect others or bringing something like COVID-19 home. But I feel like it's just an attempt to isolate me."[164] Her abuser also threatened to throw her out onto the street if she started coughing. She fears that if she leaves the house, her husband will lock her out.

Research is also beginning to indicate that the kind of violence women are experiencing in their homes during the pandemic is intensifying. More callers than usual are reporting that their partner tried to strangle or choke them. This is alarming because statistics show that attempts at strangulation in an abusive relationship means that a victim is seven times more likely to be killed by her abuser.[165]

"Instead of bruises and cuts, there are more knife wounds, strangulations, and gunshot wounds," Barbara Paradiso, director of the Center on Domestic Violence at University of Colorado Denver's School of Public Affairs, told *CU Denver News*.[166]

Ray-Jones agrees with Paradiso that women who were already in abusive situations are facing even more extreme violence. "We know that domestic violence is rooted in power and control," Ray-Jones said. "Right now, we are all feeling a lack of control over our lives, and an individual who cannot manage that will take it out on their victim."[167]

For many women, the fear of contracting the coronavirus is also preventing them from even trying to get medical care after experiencing physical abuse. "I spoke to a female caller in California that is self-quarantining for protection from COVID-19 due to having asthma," an advocate at the National Domestic Violence Hotline said. "Her partner strangled her tonight. While talking to her, it sounded like she had some really serious injuries. She is scared to go to the ER due to fear around catching COVID-19."[168]

The current crisis is making it difficult for victims and survivors to seek and get any kind of help. As hospitals and medical facilities across the country reach the breaking point, it's almost impossible for women to access medical care or therapy. Women's shelters are also dealing with overcrowding during the pandemic, and many close if the risk of infection is too high. COVID-related travel restrictions also limit women's ability to leave their abusers.[169]

Although the rise of domestic violence during COVID is not unique to America, the issue of abusers getting their hands on firearms easily is as American as apple pie. Rising right alongside COVID infection rates in America were gun sales that surged to record numbers in 2020. By the end of September 2020, it was reported that year-to-date gun sales had already surpassed those for all of 2019.[170]

Despite many gun stores closing at the beginning of the pandemic, they were later deemed "essential businesses" in many states and stayed open. This trend in gun sales is a huge red flag because studies already show that the presence of a gun in a household with a history of domestic violence makes it *five times* more likely that a woman will be murdered.[171]

Lauren Footman is the director of outreach and equity for the Coalition to Stop Gun Violence. She says in America, domestic violence and gun violence are deeply linked. Over half of all intimate partner homicides are committed with guns. Roughly four and a half million women in the United States have been threatened with a gun, and almost one million women have been shot, or shot at, by an intimate partner.[172]

As with many of the health issues discussed so far, structural racism is also at play. The CDC reports that Black and Native American women are at an increased risk for domestic violence in addition to dying from COVID-19. "There is a critical need for community-based, culturally specific organizations that specifically serve communities of color to be a part of the response to these public health crises," Footman said.[173]

Domestic violence organizations also point to a disturbing trend in their call records of initial increases followed by significant dips. Experts say this is an indication that many survivors are facing the threat of continued or escalating violence and are unable to find the space or time away from an abuser to reach out for help. Many women were out of hope and out of options.[174]

This was the case at several Asian American domestic violence organizations that provide resources for domestically abused women where staff say they felt "horror"[175] as communication with clients went quiet. After lockdown, women were pleading with staff not to call to check on them out of fear of recrimination by their abusers. In lockdown, not only were partners watching victims around the clock, but many took away their phones, cars, and credit cards, making it harder for those women to get help or leave.[176]

Women's rights advocates say that in the United States, cultural factors often prevent Asian American women from seeking help. They are the least likely group to report domestic abuse because domestic violence is often viewed as deeply stigmatizing in Asian communities. Women can face strong cultural pressures to conceal abuse and remain in violent marriages.

"There is this notion that this is our dirty laundry," Bindu Oommen-Fernandes, executive director of Narika, a domestic violence organization in California that offers multilingual help to women, told NBC News. "If a woman does leave, community members might ask: 'Why couldn't you stay? Did you have to separate and cause chaos for your children?'"[177]

After lockdowns eased in the summer of 2020, calls for help surged as Asian American women reported increased abuse during the pandemic. Experts saw another spike as fears of another lockdown in the fall or winter prompted women to flee abusive situations when they had the chance.[178]

Kavita Mehra is the executive director of Sakhi for South Asian Women, a domestic violence organization that serves immigrants in New York City. She says 166 women called the organization for help in January 2020, but by March, as New York went into quarantine, that number dropped to fifty-three calls. By April 2020, calls to the organization again started rising, and by June the number had reached 224, surpassing pre-pandemic levels.[179]

"Prior to the onset of the COVID-19 pandemic in New York City, many of the survivors that Sakhi works with were in the process of rebuilding their lives, including their financial security, in their healing process," Mehra told me. "Of the survivors that work, 90 percent of them were hourly waged workers, and from the moment that shelter-in-place orders took into effect in NYC, most survivors lost their income. As a result, survivors were facing unprecedented economic challenges that are causing severe forms of food, housing, and utility insecurity. At Sakhi, we have made an active effort to support our community at this time, and in 2020, our team distributed over $130,000 in emergency assistance and over 18,000 [pounds] of fresh food to survivors across NYC."[180]

Mehra says many immigrant women speak little English and have no family or friends in the United States, leaving them completely dependent on their partners. A lot of these women in New York also lived in COVID-19 hot spots, such as Queens and Brooklyn. Many Asian American women also face compounding factors such as racism and threats of deportation, and Mehra points out that abusive partners often use the immigration status of their victims as a form of power and control, since women cannot report abuse to the police if they are undocumented.

In an interview, Mehra told me that the pandemic has been disastrous on people's finances and created a real lack of financial security. She pointed out that the survivors are not getting the stimulus checks, and money is often a huge point of contention, and control, in abusive relationships. Mehra said organizations like hers had to step in where the government left off.

"It is clear that while we have been trying to manage the public health crisis through COVID-19, a second crisis of gender-based violence has continued to rise across our communities," Mehra said. "And it has been local, community-based organizations like Sakhi that have had to support survivors at a time when other resources have not been available. Our role as essential workers has never been more clear."[181]

The fear of getting sick from COVID prevents many survivors from even trying to leave, Mehra said. She recalled the story of a mother who stayed home while violence against her escalated. She was more scared of exposing herself and her children to the virus if she left than she was of the abuse if she stayed.

"She continued to experience violence because of her fear," Mehra said in an interview with NBC, noting that her organization helps transport survivors to a friend's or family's house. Eventually, the woman decided that the risk of life-threatening abuse outweighed her fear of contracting COVID. As a result, Sakhi paid an Uber driver to whisk the mother and her children to safety with relatives in a neighboring state.[182]

Rising anti-Asian racism tied to blaming COVID on China and Asian people is also proving to be a big barrier to leaving an abusive situation. More than 2,500 Asian Americans reported incidents of discrimination or racism in 2020 during the pandemic, according to the group Stop AAPI (Asian American and Pacific Islander) Hate. The organization says many women may fear leaving an abusive home, worrying they may be subject to racist hate crimes, retaliation for spreading a "Chinese virus."[183] While all women in abusive relationships face elevated risks of violence during the pandemic, the rise in anti-Asian racism and xenophobia has created specific challenges for AAPI survivors and the organizations that work with them.

For example, a hotline operator at the Korean American Family Services said she received a call from a Korean immigrant who had left her violent abuser but still remained unsafe even after moving to a new apartment.[184] She said her landlord had been harassing her since the pandemic started, but now he was threatening to evict her in order to prevent coronavirus from spreading in the building. It didn't matter that she was healthy. For the landlord, her ethnicity alone marked her as a contagion.

Across the country, domestic violence organizations that work with AAPI survivors report a surge in hotline calls and an unprecedented demand for support services. According to the executive director of the Korean American Family Service Center, the organization saw a 300 percent increase in call volume between March and May 2020 and continues to see twice the volume of calls seen this time last year.[185]

Experts say that even before the pandemic, AAPI survivors were less likely to report abuse and access mental health services than women of other races. Coronavirus-fueled racism compounds the alienation and invisibility of AAPI survivors. Many women may even feel safer staying with their abusers when the alternative could expose them not only to a deadly virus but also people blaming their ethnicity for it.[186]

"The amount of fear and isolation that someone feels in an abusive relationship is beyond anyone's imagination and then to have to experience the additional fear of racism when you step outside of the home," Niketa Sheth, the former executive director of Womankind, the first helpline for Asian domestic violence survivors on the East Coast, told the publication *Hyphen*.[187] She said that some of the organization's clients even experience racism and anti-Asian sentiment from the police. "You're not quite safe anywhere," Sheth said. "You are not safe at home [and] you are not safe outside of the home."[188]

Mehra told me that the pandemic has reinforced the role of people who work with survivors as essential workers. She says she is hopeful seeing the way nonprofits have come together to work cooperatively, and not against each other.

"Leaders across the sector have been facing similar challenges during the COVID-19 pandemic, which has ranged from ensuring the economic health of our respective organization to continuing to support staff during this trying time," Mehra said. "In my experience, I have seen fellow executive directors coming together to work through these challenges, either through leadership groups or deepening partnerships, to help alleviate the isolation often felt in the work."

The rise of violence against women during COVID is not only a threat in American homes. One in three women worldwide experiences physical or sexual violence, usually from an intimate partner, and since the outbreak of COVID-19, emerging data and reports all show that domestic violence has intensified. The United Nations calls it the "shadow pandemic" growing amid COVID.[189]

In Europe, one country after another seems to have followed the same pattern of a rise in domestic violence with lockdowns. First, we saw governments impose lockdowns without making sufficient, or any, provisions for domestic abuse victims. Roughly two weeks later, statistics show distress calls spike, setting off a public outcry, followed by governments scrambling to find solutions.

This pattern first manifested itself in Italy. Their lockdown began in early March 2020. Soon after that, domestic violence reports began to rise, but there was nowhere for abused women to go. Shelters could not take them because the risk of infection was too great. The Italian government told local authorities to requisition hotel rooms to serve as makeshift shelters where victims could quarantine safely.[190]

The Italian Ministry of Health, citing data from national statistics agency I.STAT, said calls to domestic violence hotlines shot up during the lockdown, registering a 75 percent increase compared to the same period in 2019. Between March and June 2020, calls and text messages to the antiviolence number more than doubled during the same period, to 119.6 percent.[191]

"Because of the restrictions, we involuntarily created profound distress that led to increased episodes of domestic violence and femicide," Prime Minister Giuseppe Conte said during a November 2020 parliamentary discussion on Italy's long-standing crisis of violence against women.[192]

In December 2020, the *New England Journal of Medicine* issued a report stating that the "pandemic has highlighted how much work needs to be done to ensure that people who experience abuse can continue to obtain access to support, refuge and medical care when another public health disaster hits."[193] The journal said that clinicians, public health officials, and policymakers all have a responsibility to increase their efforts to "address the layers of social inequalities exacerbating abuse in their communities now and moving forward."[194]

Researching domestic violence data amid COVID and reading women's stories keeps me awake at night. I think about all the ways this pandemic permeates women's lives—from our mental health to our physical safety. Quarantining might be one of the most effective strategies against this virus, but as the world went into lockdown, no government considered what violence could occur when women and children were sequestered with an abusive partner.

Sometimes I think about how two decades of working on women's health and rights has hardened me. I can discuss, dispassionately, some of the most harrowing aspects of feminist issues. But writing about the violence women are experiencing in their homes around the world and how COVID is further entrapping them with their abusers gave me nightmares.

While the misogynist administration of Donald Trump blocked

the reauthorization of the Violence Against Women Act (VAWA), kept immigrant women experiencing domestic violence from getting help, and even opposed a United Nations Security Council resolution to end rape as a weapon of war, I believe there is a lot to be hopeful for under the Biden-Harris administration.

Feminists already know that the issue of violence against women will be of utmost importance, because then senator Biden was one of the original sponsors and strongest advocates for VAWA. Not only did he spearhead the act, but he still calls it the "legislative accomplishment of which I am most proud."[195]

VAWA was signed into law in 1994, and is widely credited with helping change the way Americans understand and view domestic violence, once regarded as a "family matter"[196] that law enforcement preferred to avoid.

It was VAWA that created a national hotline for victims, funded shelters and crisis centers, and trained law enforcement in communities across the country so that they were better prepared to investigate incidents and support survivors. According to the US Department of Justice's Bureau of Justice Statistics, after VAWA passed, the overall rate of intimate partner violence declined by 64 percent from 1994 to 2010.[197]

As senator, Biden continued to lead efforts to renew and strengthen VAWA in 2000, 2005, and 2013, expanding protections to include immigrant women, rural women, Native American women, and LGBTQ+ people. Biden also introduced and helped pass the William Wilberforce Trafficking Victims Protection Reauthorization Act in 2008 and, as Barack Obama's vice president, he established the first White House adviser on violence against women. During his time with the Obama administration, Biden also led efforts to address campus sexual assault.[198]

During my time working as a policy analyst at the Feminist Majority Foundation, I witnessed the passion Biden has for women's rights up close. In chapter 2, I talked about working with then senator Biden closely on two global feminist pieces of legislation he championed in the US Senate—the Convention on the Elimination of All Forms of Discrimination Against Women (CEDAW) and the International Violence Against Women Act (IVAWA).

But Biden's passion to see both CEDAW and IVAWA ratified can be traced back to VAWA. The Feminist Majority has been fighting for VAWA since the early 1990s, and it was a part of the team that worked with Biden and his staff. Feminist Majority president, Ellie Smeal, closely authored language for the act with Biden. VAWA is among the legislative measures that Smeal considers part of her legacy. She played a very active role in the passage of VAWA in 1994 and in every subsequent fight for its reauthorization.

Often during office lunch breaks, we used to gather in the conference room and eat together. Smeal was known for sitting around with staff and reminiscing about being part of historic moments in American feminist history. The stories she told about working with Biden on VAWA, and what life was like for American domestic violence survivors before and after the legislation passed, stayed with me.

"Then-Senator Joe Biden's leadership was indispensable in the passage of VAWA," Smeal said in a press release. "You must change public policy and laws to change culture. Over the last 20 years, the Violence Against Women Act has done just that."[199]

Smeal also said she credits VAWA with establishing a national standard in the fight to reduce sexual assault, domestic violence, and stalking. "VAWA literally saved women's lives," Smeal said.[200]

But much work remains. The good news is that Biden has a plan for accomplishing this pledge in an ambitious platform for women's rights focused in five areas: healthcare, economic security, work and family, violence against women, and global women's rights. This includes reauthorizing VAWA, which expired in February 2019.

"As many as 1 in 3 women is the victim of gender-based violence at some point in her life, and that rate is even higher for women of color, lesbian and bisexual women, transgender individuals, and other members of vulnerable or underserved communities," President Biden tweeted on November 25, 2020. "The COVID-19 pandemic has made matters worse, creating a 'shadow pandemic' for many women and girls who are largely confined to their home with their abuser and facing economic insecurity that makes escape more difficult. Today, on the International Day for the Elimination of Violence Against Women, I reaffirm my commitment to ending this epidemic. A Biden-Harris administration will take bold action here at home and rejoin global efforts to confront gender-based violence in all its forms."[201]

Usually when politicians talk or tweet, I don't believe a word. But I have faith in Joe Biden when it comes to helping survivors of violence get the help they need because, on this issue, he has the record to prove it.

Depression, COVID, domestic violence—there is no doubt that we will be studying how this pandemic impacted women's health in America for years to come. Clare Wenham, an assistant professor of global-health policy at the London School of Economics, told *The Atlantic* that during an outbreak, there's a "distortion of health systems"[202] as everyone goes into crisis mode and resources are directed toward controlling the epidemic. She said that "things that aren't priorities"[203] inevitably get canceled.

Unfortunately, it is clear that women's health is not considered a priority even though it urgently needs to be, especially as women are disproportionately impacted by the pandemic. Experts agree that no one bears the brunt of "shifting health resources"[204] more acutely than pregnant women and their babies.

In the next chapter, I will discuss how, even though pre-COVID America was already in the midst of a maternal health crisis, this pandemic is on track for permanently changing how women give birth in America.

6

Pregnancy in a Pandemic

When I began writing this book, I wanted to focus on the state of maternal health in America. I thought it was unacceptable that women in America are the most likely to die from complications related to pregnancy or childbirth than women in any other wealthy nation. I still believe that.

After surviving childbirth in the United States, I started researching the issue more and was shocked to learn that these kinds of dangerous experiences are more the rule, not the exception. In 2018, there were seventeen maternal deaths for every 100,000 live births in the United States—a ratio more than double that of most other high-income countries. It is estimated that more than fifty thousand women suffer serious injuries or complications in childbirth each year in the United States. Complications include stroke, seizures, hemorrhage, and cardiac arrest. A majority of these are preventable.[1]

Women in the United States are 50 percent more likely to die in childbirth than their mothers, but that risk is three to four times higher for Black and Indigenous women. Black women have a death rate of 40.8 per 100,000 births, three times higher than that for white women. American Indian and Native Alaskan women have the next highest rate at 29.7 deaths per 100,000 live births, more than double the rate in white women.[2]

In one especially high-profile case in 2016, an American woman named Caroline Malatesta and her husband were awarded $16 million from Brookwood Medical Center in Birmingham, Alabama, after the couple successfully sued for medical negligence and reckless fraud.[3]

Malatesta told *Cosmopolitan* that she chose Brookwood because of their emphasis on "empowering experiences"[4] for women during natural childbirth. Instead, she was restrained and violently handled while in labor. Two nurses forcibly tried to delay her labor to the extent of pushing the crowning head of the baby back into the birth canal. The experience left Malatesta with a chronic pelvic pain condition and permanent nerve damage.

"Because of the trauma I sustained from fighting while birthing, I now suffer from a permanent and debilitating nerve condition called pudendal neuralgia," Malatesta wrote. "I grew up in a medical family. My dad is a doctor; my granddad was a doctor. Litigation, medical malpractice—it's not something we take lightly. When the nerve injury really revealed itself, I wasn't planning to file a lawsuit. I just wanted answers."[5]

Malatesta said that when she initially filed the lawsuit, she had no idea what to expect, but as the case went on and attracted coverage, other women from all over the country started sharing their own stories. Caroline Malatesta believes her successful lawsuit was a wake-up call for hospitals that don't listen to women and don't take them seriously.[6]

In another high-profile case, Ali Lowry almost died in the same Ohio hospital where she worked as a delivery nurse. As Lowry began breastfeeding her newborn son after a C-section, her vision went black. She was bleeding internally, but she wouldn't get proper help for hours. Her blood pressure had plummeted, and her husband, Shaun, reported he had "never seen so much blood."[7]

The doctor took Lowry back to surgery and removed six cups of blood but saw no active bleeding. When she still didn't improve, it became clear she needed a hysterectomy. But the hospital didn't have enough matching blood for the operation. As she was being transferred via helicopter to a different hospital, Ali went into cardiac arrest.

Doctors removed her uterus and found a lacerated artery. Had Ali stayed at the first hospital, said one physician, "she surely would have died."[8] Lowry said although she won't be able to have more children, she is grateful she survived. In her lawsuit, Lowry alleged her doctor and the hospital could have done more.

"I was definitely devastated by losing my uterus, but at the same time I was also so thankful to be alive and that my baby was OK," Lowry said in an interview to *USA Today*.[9] She and her husband sued the hospital and her doctor. They settled for an undisclosed amount.

In another case of obstetric violence that got a lot of press, Evelyn Yang, the wife of one-time Democratic presidential candidate Andrew Yang, bravely revealed in January 2020 that she is a survivor of sexual assault. The perpetrator, Robert A. Hadden, an ob-gyn in New York, is accused of abusing dozens of his patients—most of whom were pregnant.[10] After her exclusive interview, I also wrote a CNN op-ed on Yang.

She told CNN's Dana Bash about the abusive behavior that

began when Hadden started asking her inappropriate questions about her sexual activity unrelated to her pregnancy or the baby.[11]

"There was absolutely no premise for that line of questioning, and it seemed like he just wanted to hear about me talking about sex," Yang said. "What I kept sticking to was this: 'OK, so my doctor is pervy. I have a pervy doctor, but I'm going to focus on having a healthy baby,' and the idea of changing doctors was overwhelming for me."[12]

Yang says Hadden took advantage of her vulnerability since this was her first pregnancy. "The examinations became longer, more frequent, and I learned that they were unnecessary most of the time," she recalled, but she told herself, "I suppose I just need to trust him."[13]

Then when Yang was seven months pregnant, she says Hadden sexually assaulted her. "I was in the exam room, and I was dressed and ready to go," Yang recalled to CNN. "Then, at the last minute, he kind of made up an excuse. He said something about, 'I think you might need a C-section,' and he proceeded to grab me over to him and undress me and examine me internally, ungloved. I knew it was wrong. I knew I was being assaulted."[14]

Yang said she never told her husband or her family until she saw that another woman had reported the same doctor's alleged assault to the police. Yang subsequently joined legal action against him and testified before a grand jury, leading to Hadden's indictment on multiple felony sex charges. A 2016 plea deal revoked his medical license but gave no jail time. Yang then joined more than two dozen other women in suing Columbia University, its affiliated hospitals, and Hadden.[15]

Finally, in September 2020, he was charged with attacking girls and women for nearly two decades under the guise of medical examinations. Prosecutors described Hadden, sixty-two, as a "predator in a white coat,"[16] accusing him of singling out young and unsuspecting victims.

Yang's sheer courage is undeniable, but it also made me think of the unmitigated horror she went through, how hard she fought even as both medical and criminal justice institutions apparently failed her, and how fearless she is not only to share her story now but to continue to give a voice to survivors. It also made me think about how challenging it is to report obstetric violence. Look how difficult it was for Yang to get justice, despite all her privilege, education, and media connections.

What makes Yang's story, and that of the other women survivors, especially horrifying is that many of these women, including Yang herself, were pregnant during the time of their abuse and assault. Any woman can tell you how vulnerable you always feel at your ob-gyn's office—but that feeling is multiplied exponentially when you are pregnant. By any number of measures, pregnancy is one of the riskiest times—personally and statistically—of any woman's life.

"Everyone has their own Me Too story," she told CNN. "It's far too prevalent. But not everyone can tell their story. Not everyone has the audience or platform to tell their story, and I actually feel like I'm in this very privileged position to be able to do that."[17]

How are things like this happening in America? How are women in such a wealthy country, with such medical expertise, ending up with serious injuries, death, or assault during pregnancy and childbirth? It is a scandal most Americans remain unaware of.

When I first started digging and asking these questions, I was mostly coming across the stories of white women such as Malatesta and Lowry, or women already in the spotlight, like Evelyn Yang.

These were the stories that got the front-page coverage and write-ups in high-profile, glossy magazines. The incidents almost always ended in successful lawsuits or settlements. But of course, the vast majority don't.

Why should we single out maternal deaths as opposed to others? Because they don't just tell us the number of women dying in childbirth; they are also an indicator of women's overall position in society. Maternal mortality ratios tell us how well a country's healthcare system in general is functioning.[18] In America, our maternal mortality rates are a stark reminder of how little we actually value women's health.

Despite all the advances of modern obstetrics, American women's health is still declining. The United States is also one of the few countries in the world that doesn't have paid maternal or family leave. Twenty-five percent of moms return to work two weeks after giving birth.[19] This is all despite our spending more per capita on healthcare than any other country. The greatest irony to me, in my research, was that US government–funded programs had advocated, and achieved, safe motherhood in other countries around the world. Maternal deaths in Bangladesh were reduced by 40 percent between 2001 and 2010.[20] How is it that America's maternal mortality crisis is worsening while Bangladesh's is improving?

Before I could find answers to my questions, I left the Feminist Majority and the policymaking world. From 2013 to 2019, my writing career, which started as a "side hustle," was starting to generate income. I decided to go full-time with it.

But my passionate interest in maternal health only intensified. I continued to spotlight it every opportunity I got. I was getting more platforms to publish my work, and I appeared increasingly as a TV political commentator. It was an exciting time in my career.

Toward the end of 2018, I got an invitation that would pull me firmly back into the world of maternal health advocacy. When American supermodel and maternal health advocate Christy Turlington Burns asked me to moderate a panel at South by Southwest (SXSW) in the spring of 2019, I couldn't refuse.

Christy's amazing organization, Every Mother Counts (EMC), works to make pregnancy and childbirth safe for every mother everywhere. They raise awareness, invest in solutions, and mobilize action. This is an issue that's very close to Christy. She had a serious complication during the birth of her first child when she experienced postpartum hemorrhaging. Although Christy was lucky to have access to great healthcare that saved her life, the experience opened her eyes to how hemorrhages, just like hers, are the leading cause of pregnancy-related deaths worldwide—even in the United States.

"I was fortunate to have a birth center option available to me which was within a hospital," Christy told me in an interview for *Forbes* in 2013.[21] "This was an ideal scenario because I was able to have all the comforts of home with the proximity of emergency obstetric care in the event it was necessary. Most women don't know they have options. Others simply don't. Childbirth can and should be an empowering experience. I wish that for all those who choose to be mothers."[22]

Although our paths had crossed while lobbying and advocating on Capitol Hill in the past, Christy immediately supported my work when I started my freelancing career. She granted me interviews about her work for safe motherhood in Bangladesh, and I wrote about EMC's work for my columns in *Forbes Woman* and *Women in the World*.

South by Southwest is a very popular annual conference, almost more like a festival, that takes place in Austin, Texas. It celebrates the "convergence of the interactive, film, and music industries," according to its website.[23] While maternal health is not something you might expect to see featured at SXSW, this was an exciting opportunity to bring the issue to a new audience.

The EMC panel I moderated included pioneering midwife Jennie Joseph, CEO of Commonsense Childbirth, and Dr. Rebekah Gee, a physician who at the time was the secretary of health of Louisiana, alongside Christy herself. We screened EMC's documentary series, *Giving Birth in America*, after which I facilitated a conversation about the United States' maternal health crisis.

SXSW was the first time Dr. Gee, Christy, Jennie, and I shared the same stage making our case for investing in maternal health. Our chemistry onstage and off- was immediate. Christy brought us all together, and connecting with these women revived my activist soul.

While in Austin, we did an additional talk sponsored by the New York–based group Hamilton Place Strategies, and although the discussions were inspiring, it was talking to audience members afterward that excited me most. It took me back to my days on the Hill and reminded me how much I love connecting with fellow feminist advocates. It energizes me when women come together and organize.

Soon after I returned to Washington, I got an email from a major book publisher that wanted to discuss my writing a book on maternal health. The representative had seen me at the SXSW panel. Maternal health was becoming the epicenter of my work, and I was excited to dive back into that world.

A few months later, Christy, Jennie, Rebekah, and I reunited. This time, Rebekah brought us together in New Orleans for the

Louisiana Department of Health's first Maternal Mortality Summit. It was a meeting of public health professionals, providers, policymakers, and community leaders who came together to advocate for improving childbirth outcomes in the state.

Why Louisiana? While America has the highest maternal mortality rate among developed nations, more women die in Louisiana than in any other US state.[24] Rebekah moved there as the director of the state's Birth Outcomes Initiative and accumulated an impressive track record. She spearheaded a campaign to end early elective deliveries, which are nonmedically indicated early deliveries before thirty-nine weeks of gestation, which, in addition to her other efforts, led to statewide drops of more than 85 percent in early elective deliveries. Twenty-five percent of that number were reductions in infant mortality, and 10 percent in admissions to the neonatal ICU. Rebekah went on to become Louisiana's director of Medicare and Medicaid before being selected as the state's secretary of health.[25]

Louisiana governor John Bel Edwards opened the summit, and Rebekah welcomed everybody by highlighting the importance of elevating work related to racial equity and listening to patients. "The women of our society are the bedrock, the foundation," she said at the summit's opening. "No one should die in the State of Louisiana giving life."

But too many women *are* dying. In Louisiana, the death rate is 44.8 per 100,000 births. And once again, it's especially alarming for Black mothers. The rate of death for Black mothers in Louisiana is 72.6 for every 100,000 births, the same rate as North Korea.[26] That means for every white mother who dies, *four* Black mothers die from pregnancy-related complications.[27]

Rebekah was clear about what drives this disparity: racism. She pointed out that roughly 59 percent of Black maternal deaths are preventable, compared to 9 percent of white maternal deaths.[28] What Rebekah was saying shouldn't have been shocking, but hearing a white woman being so honest about the role of racism was refreshing.

"Don't blame women," Rebekah said in an interview to NOLA. com. "It's implicit bias. We all have it."[29]

Being a part of this summit changed the lens through which I viewed America's maternal health crisis. It showed me that the face of America's maternal health crisis is Black. The reality of the numbers came alive for me in Louisiana. The majority of the audience at the summit was Black women—nurses, policymakers, community leaders, doulas, and midwives. Prior to this summit, my work had been mostly on the policy side. That world in Washington, DC, is very white. And a panel on giving birth in America, at a trendy conference like SXSW, meant being surrounded again by mostly white, wealthy attendees. But Louisiana brought the role of race front and center for me.

I got to listen to woman after woman tell their stories, recounting their troubling experiences giving birth at hospitals, having their symptoms ignored, waiting for hours to be seen. Christy and I spoke at a panel where we listened to mothers tell stories of how their premature babies died in the NICU. One woman, Malika Bilal, told the story of how her sister-in-law suffered a stroke while pregnant that left her partially paralyzed.

"She kept telling them [the nurses] that her blood pressure was skyrocketing and she had a pounding migraine," Bilal told me.[30] "But no one came to help."

I was amazed at the range of the experiences women of color were reporting, especially Black women. Behind every number is a real woman, somebody's daughter, sister, partner, mother. It's easy to forget, when faced with a shocking statistic, what the numbers represent.

I also think we forget how intertwined our lives are. Why should you care about so many Black women dying? How does it impact you? Because the health of Black women is a litmus test for how much we need to invest in and prioritize women's health overall. The state of care available to women of color is a warning for all American women.

But for much of American history, health disparities between Blacks and whites were largely blamed on Black people's supposed "susceptibility to illness,"[31] or what one doctor in 1903 called their "mass of imperfections."[32] These gaps in health were framed as an African American problem, when they were in fact an American problem.

Social scientists and medical researchers increasingly agree that racism is driving the disparities, not race. A 2016 analysis of five years of data even found that Black, college-educated mothers who gave birth in local hospitals were more likely to suffer severe complications of pregnancy or childbirth than white women who never graduated from high school.[33]

In Louisiana, I found the answer to my burning question of why everyone in America wasn't talking about the scandal of our maternal health crisis—because it was mostly Brown and Black women who were dying. It explained why there was so little national outrage over it.

Another speaker at the summit was Britain's famous Dr. Gwyneth Lewis, the former national clinical leader for maternity services for the United Kingdom's National Health Service. She is widely credited with successfully driving down maternal mortality rates in the United Kingdom. During the 1950s, the United States and the

United Kingdom had the same rate of women dying in pregnancy and childbirth, but now Britain's rate is almost three times lower.[34]

Dr. Lewis told the audience that it would be more effective to frame America's maternal health crisis as a women's health crisis because "no one would care about a Black women's health crisis." I was shocked that an elderly white woman was bold enough to make such a statement to a largely Black audience. Even though I knew Dr. Lewis was right, it seemed borderline offensive to say out loud.

But that was in 2019, in a pre-COVID world. Today, when I look back to that moment, I think about how bold white women like Dr. Lewis and Rebekah were to be calling out something that the COVID pandemic has made obvious and undeniable. What's killing American women in childbirth? Systemic racism, or to put it more politely, "implicit bias."

The intersection of gender and race puts the lives of women of color especially at risk, and in the United States, where childbirth was already the number one reason people are admitted to the hospital, the pandemic made a bad situation even worse for pregnant women.[35]

Dr. Rachael Overcash is an attending physician specializing in maternal and fetal medicine at MedStar Washington Hospital Center in DC. MedStar is a not-for-profit healthcare organization operating more than 120 entities, including ten hospitals in the Washington, DC, area. She told me in an interview that at the start of the pandemic, there was a lot of fear, and the medical field was uncertain about the management of COVID.

"There were a lot of mixed messages about best practice and protocols," Dr. Overcash said.[36] People were focused on controlling the spread of the virus, making room for a surge of COVID patients, postponing elective surgeries, rationing out limited masks, scrambling around shortages in basic personal protective equipment (PPE), etc.

As images of overwhelmed hospitals—stretched thin with a crippling virus—and dying patients flooded the front pages of newspapers, American hospitals became battlefields. Policies in healthcare administration changed overnight with telehealth rather than in-person consultations. Universal masking was required, and patients who did go to a hospital for consultation faced the risk of contracting the virus. Women no longer knew whether their birth partners, companions, or even their doctors would be attending their delivery. Many women had no option.

Betty Islinger never thought she would have to give birth alone. Because of the pandemic, she went into labor and gave birth with no one she knew by her side.

"I was one of the terrified pregnant women you have been hearing about during this pandemic who were told they could only bring one person to the hospital," she recalled.[37] "Before the pandemic, I had big plans for my partner, my mother, and even a doula to be a part of my support system as I brought another child into the world. The closer I got to my due date, all that went out the window!"

Islinger says she packed food for herself and ended up going to the hospital alone. "My multipage birth plan zeroed in on just making it out of the hospital safe and fast."

Parveen Phillips went into labor a month after America went into lockdown and was becoming increasingly anxious watching the scenes of hospitals at their breaking point across the country. Phillips tried to move up her scheduled C-section, but the hospital was booked. Her impending due date started to feel increasingly scary. She was informed that her husband would not be allowed to be with her.

When Phillips delivered, she was alone and her baby was immediately taken away from her while doctors awaited Parveen's COVID test results. "I didn't even get to see what she looked like," Phillips recalled.[38] After learning she was negative, Phillips was allowed to breastfeed her baby, but she had to wear a mask.

Two days later, Phillips was discharged from the hospital and allowed to go home. "The entire experience was really scary," she said. "I know everyone is doing their best. We are all in unknown territory. But it is so traumatic giving birth without your partner, or somebody to support you as you are bringing this new life into the world. Can you imagine giving birth alone, scared, with a mask on? Just being in a hospital was terrifying."

In the early days of the pandemic, women also had to deal with conflicting information from health agencies. Should newborns be immediately isolated from their mothers? Should early breastfeeding be avoided? While the CDC in the United States recommended temporary separation, the WHO recommended the opposite—putting babies with their infected mothers in the same room.

Ava Letterman was heavily pregnant with her second child, with a due date in early May, several months into lockdown. Everything was going fine despite all the precautions and regulations that had been put in place. Letterman says her biggest worry at the time was that she wouldn't be able to have her husband by her side.

When she went into labor a few weeks later, restrictions had loosened at the hospital and Letterman was allowed to have her partner with her. "The nurse and all the staff had their masks on, but otherwise everything felt normal," Letterman said.

When she was told they'd need to test her for coronavirus, as per new hospital regulations, she agreed to a swab test. Letterman says the test was uncomfortable and her contractions were becoming more intense, but then the energy in the room suddenly changed.

"I could see them whispering, but I was exhausted and in pain, so I wasn't really focusing on what they were saying," Letterman recalled.[39] Then her doctor came in and told her she had tested positive for COVID.

Letterman held on to her husband's hand. She was terrified. How could this have happened? She had no symptoms and no idea how she got infected. She hadn't even left her house for the entire last month of the pregnancy. Letterman felt overwhelmed with guilt.

"I was paranoid that everyone in the hospital was judging me," she said. "I was convinced they thought I wouldn't be a good mother and that I was reckless for getting COVID. I kept apologizing." Anyone who came into Letterman's room had to be in full PPE, and as her labor got underway, she said all she was thinking about was getting her baby out safely in the world. "I even forgot I tested positive."

Letterman said when she was discharged from the hospital, they sent her home without much information about her having COVID, so she stayed indoors and self-isolated with her baby.

"Those first few days were hard," she said. "I struggled a lot. I felt scared to tell anyone I knew about my positive test. It was embarrassing."

The chaos brought on by the pandemic is pushing maternity care, and women's needs, further down on the list of health priorities, and women are feeling it. A 2020 study by Elizabeth Mollard at the University of Nebraska Medical Center and Amaya Wittmaack from the University of Virginia School of Medicine found that pregnant women felt less supported during their childbirth experience due to the changes in maternity unit practices related to the pandemic. More than a fifth of the women reported feeling unsafe in the maternity unit, and more than 60 percent of the women in the study said they did not receive adequate support during childbirth.[40]

"Healthcare policy and maternity care practices should focus not only on keeping women safe from COVID-19 infection but also on ways to increase women's overall feelings of safety and control in their birthing environment," the study concluded. "In declaring hospitals to be safe for delivery, the patient's emotional safety in a highly stressed situation such as childbirth must also be ensured."[41]

But a year into the pandemic, pregnant women are still not a priority. Dr. Overcash said that initially experts did not know if pregnant women were at higher risk of contracting the COVID virus; however, subsequent data showed they did not have a higher chance of being infected. Early in the pandemic, MedStar started testing all women admitted in labor.

"Knowing if someone was COVID positive or not provided a lot of reassurance to frontline providers caring for women," she said. "It also allowed us to monitor closer infants born to COVID-positive women to see if they developed any symptoms."

As study after study shows us, when things are bad for white women in America, they are worse for women of color, and even worse for Black women. Dr. Overcash described to me the acute impact the pandemic is having on Latina women in Washington, DC, who tend to live in multigenerational homes. What she is seeing is consistent with the CDC, which finds that nationwide Hispanic or Latina mothers make up nearly half of the coronavirus cases among pregnant women.

Maybe Americans had the luxury of ignoring or debating the role of race in the quality of healthcare people received before COVID. But the pandemic is making race an undeniable factor in who survives the pandemic, and nowhere did this reality play out more clearly than with maternal health in New York City, the epicenter of COVID in the United States.

Research confirms that people of color are more likely than white people to be exposed to COVID-19, require hospitalization, and die. But even pre-pandemic, racial disparities in healthcare in New York were already stark. The racialized impacts of COVID showed up from day one, and now it is a confirmed fact that Black and Latino New Yorkers are dying at double the rate of white people.

"Disparities in care became crystal clear during the pandemic," Sascha James-Conterelli, president of the New York State Association of Licensed Midwives and a chairwoman of the state's task force on maternal mortality and disparate racial outcomes, said in an interview with Yale's School of Nursing. "Hospitals in the middle of boroughs, where populations are predominantly non-white, were the last to get PPE and point-of-care testing, but they had the greatest number of people affected by the virus."[42]

Once again, women's health is hit harder. While Black women were already three to four times more likely to die of childbirth-related causes than white women, in New York City, they are *eight to twelve* times more likely to die. James-Conterelli says that to see those numbers graphed on a daily basis demonstrated the undeniable racial disparities.[43]

"Pregnant women were dying in those hospitals because there were barriers to being tested and barriers to being protected," she said.[44] James-Conterelli explains that while the reasons why pregnant and birthing women die are essentially the same around the world, in the United States, the issue of racism is an additional factor.

"When we really look at the bottom line, yes, access to care is an issue," she said. "However, a bigger issue is the fact that even when you have a well-educated Black person with access to care and means and money—this population is dying at an even higher rate than less-educated, lower-income, more marginalized folks."[45]

James-Conterelli cites the example of tennis legend Serena Williams, who suffered life-threatening complications after the birth of her daughter in 2017. Williams had shortness of breath and, as a professional athlete, knew something was wrong with her body. But Williams's requests for a CT scan and blood thinner were repeatedly ignored by medical staff, who assured her that her pain medication was making Williams "confused."[46] When a CT scan was finally ordered it showed that several small blood clots had settled in Williams's lungs.

James-Conterelli points out that even the symptoms of a rich and famous Black woman like Williams, who is in peak physical condition and has access to the best medical care, can still be ignored. This proves that nothing protects Black women from the color of their own skin.[47]

"It must be racism," James-Conterelli said. "There is nothing else, because when you start to drill down and really look at case-by-case scenarios, you see subtle holes in care that if it's taken in one instance, it may not be anything, but when you line it all up, you will realize there is a huge systemic problem of how people view Black people, regardless of income, education, or socio-economic status."[48]

The role of racism in women's healthcare may have been brought into sharp focus because of the pandemic, but in the early days of COVID there was chaos everywhere. For example, New York City hospitals were quick to implement the "one-person policy" where only one person was allowed to attend a birth, making pregnant women choose between family members and increasing their isolation. Some hospitals were not allowing anyone, doulas or spouses, to be present during labor or birth.

But this policy disproportionately impacted women of color, especially Black women who are more likely to hire a doula, a person who is employed to provide guidance and support to a pregnant woman during labor. Several studies have shown that having a doula or other support person present during birth can improve outcomes for birthing people and their babies.

Jamarah Amani, a midwife and the director of the Southern Birth Justice Network, said in an interview that doulas are especially important for Black patients and other women of color who experience discrimination during birth. "Having an advocate there can be lifesaving," she told *Vox*.[49] Amani says doulas can be instrumental in getting the right medication or being heard about the symptoms or pain level. "Doulas, for many marginalized people, are essential," Amani said. "They're essential workers."[50]

Monica McLemore is an American nurse and an associate professor of family health nursing at the University of California, San Francisco. She thinks the unfortunate reality of the coronavirus pandemic is that it showed us how unprepared and underfunded the public health infrastructure in the United States is to address the basic needs of its citizens.

McLemore's article in *Scientific American*, "COVID-19 Is No Reason to Abandon Pregnant People," was an early warning about how strategies like the one-person policy, intended to conserve personal protective equipment and slow the spread of COVID, don't consider the impact on women of color.[51]

"The recent decision of some of the city's hospitals should raise concern about how the barring of doulas and spouses may disproportionately affect populations, such as Black women, who are already vulnerable to disbelief and mistreatment by hospital staff—a situation that could potentially worsen without anyone there to advocate for them," she wrote.[52]

McLemore told me in an interview that COVID laid bare many of the inequities in healthcare in the United States. She said that as she reflects now on the piece she wrote in 2020 at the height of the pandemic surge in New York City, she still stands by every word.[53]

"Surviving a pandemic requires a collective effort," she said. "Ensuring those most vulnerable in our society receive the support they need is an ethical imperative. To suggest that birthing people be isolated from the essential support they need as they bring new people into the world should be considered only as a last resort."

As the pandemic continues and some hospitals reversed such policies, other hospitals around the country continue to limit birthing people to one support person. Experts say it's important to know the rules and regulations of your specific hospital but that might not be enough to make pregnant women less anxious—especially for women of color.

A study published in 2020 in the medical journal *Obstetrics & Gynecology* found that New York's racial disparities cannot be blamed solely on hospital quality. It reports that even when Black and Latina women gave birth in the same New York City hospitals as white women, and had similar insurance, they were still more likely to experience more life-threatening complications than white mothers.[54]

The study found that across New York, the risk of a near-death experience was 52 percent higher for Black mothers and 44 percent higher for Latinas than white women, regardless of insurance and after adjusting for other risk factors, such as diabetes and hypertension.[55]

As the city was ravaged by the pandemic in early 2020, the deaths of two Black women in childbirth garnered national attention, putting the spotlight on how no one is paying a higher price for America's maternal health crisis than Black women. One of those women was twenty-six-year-old Amber Isaac. She had tried to switch to a home or birth-center delivery after failing to get an in-person appointment with her obstetrician as providers switched to telemedicine in the wake of the shutdown.[56]

Isaac knew her platelet levels—which help blood clot—had started to drop. But because of the pandemic, her routine doctor's visits turned into Zoom conference calls, where she answered a few screening questions. Isaac got updated blood work because she decided she wanted to hire a doula or midwife for an at-home delivery during the pandemic, partially because she felt so neglected by her hospital. But she was labeled too high-risk for an out-of-hospital birth and was told she needed a surgeon after discovering her platelet counts were still falling.[57]

Isaac tried to raise the alarm and figure out what was happening with her pregnancy, but her medical team at first ignored her calls. When she finally had blood work done and was later admitted to the hospital, she entered scared and alone—neither her mother nor her partner were allowed to join her.[58]

"Can't wait to write a tell all about my experience during my last two trimesters dealing with incompetent doctors" at a Bronx hospital, Isaac wrote about the care she was getting at the hospital in a tweet on April 17, 2020, that went viral.[59] Four days later, she died after being induced more than a month early and then rushed into an emergency C-section. The surgeon she had been assigned wasn't present.

Bruce McIntyre, Isaac's partner, says she advocated for herself over and over again but was ignored. "All of this was 100 percent preventable," McIntyre told the *Guardian* in an interview.[60] "All of it. I feel like she would have got more attentive care if she was a white mother, to be completely honest with you."

Angela D. Aina, interim executive director of the Black Mamas Matter Alliance, agrees. "Implicit bias, racism, being very dismissive of people that look like Amber, making assumptions," she said, "this is the result."[61]

Isaac gave birth to a baby boy, Elias, and McIntyre is raising him. "It's very hard being in this home and imagining her here with us," McIntyre said. "She never got to even meet him. She never got to see him. And she was just so thrilled about having him."[62]

Another woman whose death gained nationwide attention was Sha-Asia Washington. She died in childbirth after going to a Brooklyn hospital for a routine stress test, a few days past her due date. After some observation, doctors noticed her blood pressure was high and gave Washington Pitocin, a drug to induce labor.[63]

But when Washington went into labor, she was asked if she wanted an epidural, something she was hesitant about, but she eventually gave in to her doctors. It was clear she was going to need a cesarean delivery. However, Washington went into cardiac arrest while her baby was delivered via C-section. Doctors spent forty-five minutes trying to save her with CPR, but she died on the table. Her newborn daughter, Khloe, was healthy.[64]

Experts and advocates point to an increase in C-sections during the pandemic, after years of advocacy campaigns against this major invasive surgery. "They were giving her too much medication," Jasmin Lopez, the sister of Washington's partner, told reporters.[65] "She said she didn't want [the epidural], and they forced it on her."

News of Washington's death spread on social media, and more than one hundred protesters showed up to demonstrate outside the hospital. "Black birthing people are already more likely to die, regardless of their income or education," Dr. Joia Crear-Perry, an obstetrician and president of the National Birth Equity Collaborative, a nonprofit dedicated to eliminating racial disparities in birth outcomes, told the *New York Times*.[66] "Now, with Covid, resources are scarce and hospitals don't have what they need. Who bears the brunt? The people least likely to be listened to."

But as research has shown, even Black women with better socioeconomic backgrounds than both Washington and Isaac, or with more educational degrees, are not any safer. The pandemic is making that clear, too.

After complications from preeclampsia, Dr. Chaniece Wallace, a chief pediatric resident at the Indiana University School of Medicine in Indianapolis, died. Four days earlier, she had given birth prematurely by cesarean delivery. Her daughter, Charlotte Wallace, was born weighing four and a half pounds, so the medical team moved her to the neonatal intensive care unit.[67]

Dr. Wallace's husband, Anthony Wallace, told her story on a GoFundMe page: "On October 20th, 2020 [Chaniece's] doctors informed us that she was developing symptoms of preeclampsia." He added that she had a ruptured liver and high blood pressure and that her kidney function was declining. "Chaniece fought with every piece of strength, courage, and faith she had available."[68]

In announcing Dr. Wallace's death, Riley Children's Hospital wrote that "it is with grievous and broken hearts that we announce the loss of one of our beloved friends, colleagues, and co-chiefs."[69] The hospital explained that she "suffered postpartum complications after delivering a healthy 35wk baby girl. [S]he received excellent care at her delivery hospital by a complete and equally devastated healthcare team."[70]

Women physicians, though, weren't convinced by the hospital's statement because of the grim statistics that bore out the dispro-portionate rate at which Black women are dying in childbirth in the United States. They went on social media to highlight how Dr. Wallace's death was indicative of the fact that Black, Native Ameri-can, and Alaska Native women are two to three times more likely to die from pregnancy-related causes than white women.[71] COVID is only spotlighting what we already know to be true.

Dr. Rachel Vreeman, a white physician, tweeted: "Heart-broken over a new loss: a female pediatrician at a great academic medical center, with the same terrible pregnancy complication that I had. Except she is Black and she died."[72]

In November 2020, Black women in Congress began to take action, sounding the alarm around COVID and maternal health in America. On the House of Representatives floor, Representative Alma Adams (D-NC) addressed the crisis and its disproportionate impact on communities that already face racial health disparities.[73]

"What we do know is that before the pandemic, Black and Brown mothers were already dying at alarming and unacceptable rates," Adams, founder and cochair of the Black Maternal Health Caucus, said in an interview to *Essence*. "In particular, Black women from all walks of life were three to four times more likely to die from pregnancy-related complications than white women. . . . We are facing a crisis within a crisis."[74]

Along with Adams, fellow members of the Congressional Black Caucus (CBC), including Representative Robin Kelly, Representative Lauren Underwood, Representative Ayanna Pressley, Representative Sheila Jackson Lee, and Representative Karen Bass, chair of the CBC, have been working with stakeholders and with Vice President Kamala Harris to develop legislation and plans for eliminating maternal health disparities.[75]

Last summer, now vice president Harris and Adams also co-sponsored the COVID-19 Bias and Anti-Racism Training Act. The legislation is aimed at ensuring hospitals and healthcare providers involved in COVID-19 testing, treatment, vaccine distribution, and response receive implicit-bias training.[76]

And yet, there are still no shortages to the stories of Black women dying in childbirth, 60 percent of which are preventable, according to the CDC.[77] If anything, the pandemic is making an already bad situation worse, but it is also highlighting that when women of color enter the medical system, they are often reduced to their race—and all the discrimination that comes with it.

I can't stop thinking about Arika Samantha Trim. Her body was flown back to her native Tobago after she died in June 2020, one week after giving birth by emergency C-section to a baby boy at thirty and a half weeks.[78]

Trim was a dedicated public servant who served in the Obama administration, both in the office of First Lady Michelle Obama and at the US Department of Agriculture. She then went on to work in the House of Representatives' Committee on Education and Labor.[79]

At the time of her death, Trim was serving at the American Hospital Association, where her job was to communicate the critical needs of the nation's hospitals during the COVID-19 pandemic. She was passionate about school nutrition and ensuring that every person has access to affordable healthcare.[80]

We have to remember and tell these stories of the women behind the statistics. Behind every one of these numbers is a real woman with real dreams. Their lives matter. Every woman's life matters. Every woman's life counts.

7

Seeking Alternatives

Why are we forcing women to give birth in overwhelmed hospitals during a pandemic? America is a country that was already in the midst of a women's health crisis, especially for women of color. Why aren't women given more options, especially now with COVID making things worse? Why is hospital birth presented as the safest, best, and only choice for most women when it is clearly not? If there's ever a time to review this line of thinking, it's now, during this pandemic. Women need safer options than giving birth in hospitals.

Many Black women were already turning to out-of-hospital births pre-COVID.[1] Now, with concerns around exposure to COVID, and existing data on systemic racism killing women in maternity wards across the country, even more women are choosing not to give birth in hospitals.

Kiki Jordan, a certified nurse-midwife, said she's received a lot more calls from Black expectant mothers during the pandemic. "COVID hit right around the same time that lots of people were starting to talk, and there was a lot of awareness gained about outcomes for Black women and Black babies in the hospitals," Jordan told Marketplace.[2] "The combination of those two things— definitely we've seen people actually taking the leap and choosing out-of-hospital birth. It's been like nothing I've ever seen before."

Dr. Joia Crear-Perry explains that in America, we equate hospitals with protection. "In the US we have dictated safety to mean the highest level of technology," she said in an interview with *Vox*.[3] "But when it comes to birthing, the evidence shows us that what makes us safe is actually being heard and listened to and valued."

She thinks that access to Black practitioners and others "who represent the communities they care for,"[4] whether they are midwives, nurses, or ob-gyns, is critical. Experts back Dr. Crear-Perry. A 2019 study found that Black patients got better care when they saw Black providers,[5] and a 2021 study showed that the mortality rate was cut in half when Black babies were cared for after their birth by doctors of the same race.[6]

"I have said for years that birthing people deserve a wider range of birthing options than hospital-based birth," Monica McLemore told me in an interview. "Major investments need to be made in birth centers and home birth, including the spaces to make this happen, funding for education and training, respectful payment models, and frankly the appreciation that normal physiologic birth is just that, a process to be witnessed, not a disease state to be managed."

For Sophia Rogers, twenty-nine, avoiding the risk of infection from the virus and unnecessary medical interventions were major reasons she decided to have a home birth. Rogers was already having issues with her OB and felt that she was constantly repeating herself to providers who were changing hands all the time. "I felt like they couldn't care less about my well-being," Rogers said. "No one asked me how I was feeling."[7]

In December 2020, Rogers delivered her son at home in Ashburn, Virginia, with her husband, Paul, following a twenty-nine-hour labor supervised by a midwife. "They definitely would have given me a C-section if I had gone to the hospital," Rogers told me. "And who knows if I would have gotten to meet my baby? So many Black mothers don't."

Misha Hylton says there were two reasons she didn't want to give birth to her first child at a hospital in the middle of COVID. "The first reason was that everything was so chaotic because of the pandemic," she said.[8] "And the second reason was because I am a woman of color. And to be honest, that scared me more than COVID."

Like Rogers, Hylton said the statistics of Black maternal deaths, even pre-pandemic, combined with her concerns about getting infected with COVID in the hospital, were enough to make her seek out a midwife. Hylton gave birth to a healthy baby girl at home, with her husband and mother present with her.

Courteney Brown was about twenty-six weeks pregnant when her doctor told her that her iron levels were so low, she would need regular infusion treatments. But it was March, the coronavirus pandemic was taking the United States by storm, and the last thing Brown wanted to do was go to an ER in a hospital.

Brown was able to find an outpatient center to get the infusions, where staff members were scheduling only two patients at a time. Even though she was able to get to a medical facility, she said going was extremely stressful. "I was terrified of getting infected," Brown said.[9] As the pandemic worsened, she called the center to make an appointment when she was informed they were closing because of COVID. The nurse on the phone told Brown to just go to the ER.

"I couldn't believe what this woman was saying," Brown said. "I am pregnant and high-risk. Why would she want to send me to an ER full of people with COVID symptoms? Did she not care if I got infected?"

Brown was convinced the lack of compassion the nurse had toward her was because of the color of her skin. It was a critical moment for Brown. She got off the phone and told her husband, "We have to make other arrangements for me to give birth safely."

She found a nearby birthing center and hired a midwife. That summer, Brown delivered her son with her husband by her side. "This center was so different from being in a hospital," Brown said. "I cannot believe the respect and love I was given."

Feeling supported was also a priority for Brittany Dandy when she learned she was expecting in March. "I was pregnant for the first time, there's a worldwide pandemic, New York City health care is completely falling apart and every headline I read is specifically about Black women, maternal health and COVID," she said in an interview with the nonprofit news organization, Marketplace.[10] "I knew that I needed to advocate for myself, more than other women."

Dandy also had to consider the price. Even with insurance, labor and delivery cost an average of $4,500 out of pocket. And not all insurance plans cover at-home births, which cost anywhere between $4,000 and $8,000. In the end, Dandy's plan did cover a home birth, so she got in touch with a midwife in Brooklyn. Even though the center was having to turn away women who were nearing labor, Kimm Sun, the owner, took Dandy in as a patient. "If you are a Black woman, we are going to prioritize you first because we know that it's going to be harder for you to get help," Sun said.[11]

Advocates have been calling for greater access to nonhospital birthing options, whether at a birthing center or at home with a midwife. The pandemic is drawing enormous attention to such alternatives to combat the discrimination Black and other patients of color can face in hospital settings.

While many Americans may think of giving birth at home as unsafe, "backward," and/or scary, with COVID, there has been an increase in demand for the services of midwives and doulas among white patients. Many white women are now facing some of the same fears Black birthing people have long dealt with, such as being disregarded by hospital staff. In New York, home-birth midwives say their calendars are fully booked, a spike they say is driven in part by white women.[12]

"People are reconsidering their birth plans and doing whatever they need to avoid hospitals," Sarita Bennett, president of the Midwives Alliance of North America, said in an interview to the *Times*.[13] She trained and worked at a hospital as a physician before becoming a midwife.

She believes planned home births can be a good option for a pregnant person who is healthy and has a low risk of complications, primarily because they are less likely to be rushed into a risky medical intervention like a C-section.

"The management model in the hospital that has led to our poor outcomes is nothing more than a corporate business model, and I understand it," Bennett told *Business Insider*.[14] "That's what you have to do. Whenever you flip burgers at McDonald's, everything has to be the same and you have to control the flow. I get it. What you get in home birth is care where the care is individualized to the family, to the person."

Until her eighth month of pregnancy, Jessica Salter had not

even thought about a home birth. "I wasn't anti them," she wrote in her column in *Vogue* magazine.[15] "Several friends had given birth at home and raved about the lack of a bumpy, excruciating commute to hospital, thrilled that they could get into their own beds moments after delivering. It was just that I gravitated towards the security that a medical setting promised."

But with the pandemic raging, Salter had to reconsider. Her partner was no longer allowed to come to her appointments. That, combined with the thought of picking up the virus in a hospital and her heightened nervousness about leaving her home, convinced Salter to look into finding a midwife.[16]

"As soon as I made the booking, I felt a huge wave of relief," Salter said. "It's been a particularly strange time to be pregnant, where I've often felt fearful and anxious and uncared for by an overstretched medical system," Salter added. "In opting for a home birth, I felt like I was making a decision for myself."[17]

Salter also points out how if you are low-risk, the statistics are on your side. A report published in *The Lancet* medical journal found that out of half a million women around the world who had home births, 40 percent were less likely to need a caesarean, 50 percent were less likely to have an instrumental birth, 55 percent were less likely to have an episiotomy (an incision made in the perineum to avoid tearing), 40 percent were less likely to have a third- or fourth-degree tear, and 75 percent were less likely to contract an infection.[18]

This report came on the heels of another report from *The Lancet* in 2020 that low-risk pregnant women who give birth at home had no increased chance of the baby's perinatal or neonatal death compared to having their babies in a hospital.[19]

Like Salter, Gloria Lopez is another example of rising home births among women who are not Black. Lopez says her worst fear was having to choose who would stand by her side at the hospital when she gave birth: her partner or her birthing assistant, or doula. The Arizona hospital where she had planned her delivery warned Lopez that only one person would be allowed in the room because of new pandemic rules. But even that could change, leaving Lopez to deliver her baby alone.

"Things were changing so fast," Lopez said. "Everything was making me anxious."[20] The prospect of giving birth in a hospital alone in the middle of a pandemic terrified her. So, at forty weeks pregnant, she found a midwife and turned to a home birth.

Seeking out midwives in America is not a new trend or option, even if the pandemic is creating a surge. According to historian and certified nurse midwife Michelle Drew, midwifery has a long tradition in the United States. She says in the late nineteenth and early twentieth centuries, midwifery was the norm, and almost half of all births were attended by midwives. "Ninety percent [of midwives] were Black women, and 10% were ethnic immigrants," Drew told Marketplace.[21] "Physicians still really weren't attending births because it was not considered important."

Prior to the twentieth century, midwives were respected community-based healthcare providers with intimate knowledge of birth processes who enjoyed close relationships with their clients. As the growing medical profession grew with the rise of surgery and handwashing, doctors—predominantly white men— openly advocated for midwives to be eliminated.[22]

By the early 1900s, the movement to delegitimize midwifery rose alongside immigrant quotas and Jim Crow laws. Physicians and health officials across the country published articles linking midwifery to high rates of infant and maternal mortality, blaming Eastern European and Black women for public health emergencies with the same arguments used to blame immigrants for diseases caused by overcrowding and poor sanitation: "illiteracy, carelessness and general filth," Kennedy Austin, a degree candidate at Columbia University's Mailman School of Public Health, wrote in her February 2020 article, "End Racial Disparities in Maternal Health, Call a Midwife."[23]

In 1921, Congress passed the Sheppard-Towner Act requiring all midwives to undergo health-safety training. Although the bill aimed to minimize lethal maternal health risks, advocates mapped race and ethnicity onto hygiene and inadequate healthcare systems, creating a racist image of the midwife. "As a result, midwives were banned from hospitals, and by 1951, 90 percent of women gave birth in hospitals," according to Austin.[24]

The white male medical establishment wanted to "[elevate] the importance of obstetrics in the eyes of practitioners, medical students, and the laity," in part by calling for the "gradual abolition of midwives in large cities," according to a 1912 paper published by J. Whitridge Williams, MD, the founder of academic obstetrics in the United States.[25] He was the recognized leader of this discipline in America during the first thirty years of the twentieth century.

"They essentially demonized the midwives," Drew said. "'Why would you possibly want some dirty, old Black woman who is probably not literate, when you could have a physician?'"[26]

As birth grew increasingly medicalized in the twentieth century, physicians were aggressive about taking out their competition. They actively advocated for the elimination of "granny midwives"[27] in medical journals. In 1915, prominent obstetrician Joseph DeLee called midwifery "a relic of barbarism."[28]

"Historically, American women were served by midwives who learned their trade empirically and passed their traditional skills down through generations," Jennie Joseph, British-trained midwife, founder, and executive director of Commonsense Childbirth Inc., wrote in an Every Mother Counts blog post. "Thousands of African American midwives, especially in the South, supported and protected women through their childbearing years until the early twentieth century. A reliable and functional system was decimated as the politics of race, power, money, and control swayed women from the home to the hospital as the preferred place of birth, and began to undermine the safety of the community-based midwife as the practitioner of choice."[29]

Joseph says that physicians became interested in delivering *all* babies. Legislation was passed, and white public health nurses were dispatched to "train" the traditional midwives. Simultaneously, states began programs to "retire" them, often by trickery, in order to stop them from practicing.[30]

"This systematic dismantling of a staunch and necessary service continued over half a century," Joseph says. "Alabama, for example, finally outlawed midwifery entirely in 1976, and to this day community-based midwives are not legal in almost half the states in America."[31]

Even though in some rural parts of the South, Black midwives continued to deliver babies for poor Black and white families, sociologist Dr. Alicia D. Bonaparte wrote in her dissertation on midwives that women of color "suffered devaluation"[32] and stigmatization. They were viewed as "illegitimate medical practitioners."[33] Even today, national midwifery licensing does not exist in the United States as it does in many other countries, and a quarter of the states do not even offer midwife licenses, making the practice of home birth effectively illegal in many parts of America.[34]

Increased interest in out-of-hospital births has not translated into better access or insurance coverage, either. That means patients typically pay $300 to $1,000 out of pocket for a birth, putting the option out of reach for many low-income patients.[35]

Cost is a major barrier for poor people to access out-of-hospital births. Medicaid, the federal state health insurance program that covers many low-income pregnant women, pays for home births in only a handful of states. Since 2015, the list includes California, but reimbursement is low, and bureaucratic requirements make it difficult for most midwives to accept Medi-Cal, California's Medicaid program.[36]

The Southern Birth Justice Network and other groups focused on Black maternal health and rights are calling for comprehensive insurance coverage and other support for midwife care as one way to help Americans have better birth experiences. Advocates also say we must integrate midwives as part of birthing teams, attending births alongside obstetricians.[37]

The American College of Nurse-Midwives and the American College of Obstetricians and Gynecologists (ACOG) even released a joint statement supporting "team-based care."[38] Although models like these are common in hospitals around the world, the United States is behind.

Increasing women's birthing options does not mean we should shun hospitals. Women's health experts stipulate that home births or birthing centers are not for everyone, and some underlying conditions, like diabetes, can make home birth more dangerous. It's also not an option when a woman needs to deliver by C-section, and many women from all races feel safer giving birth in a hospital than at home.

"I don't want a home birth," Dr. Crear-Perry said in an interview with *Vox*.[39] "I had three children who were born in hospitals."

But we cannot let hospitals off the hook. What women need, in addition to greater access to out-of-hospital births, are a slate of reforms to keep Black birthing people and other patients of color safer, regardless of where they deliver.[40]

But the distrust between women of color and white medical establishments goes beyond America's maternal health crisis and the current pandemic. Like so many things that pertain to race in America, the roots of the medical system, particularly as they affect Black women, can be traced back to the days of slavery. To move forward, we must face this brutal history.

How many American women know the story of J. Marion Sims? Considered by many to be the Father of Modern Gynecology,[41] the nineteenth-century gynecologist is credited with inventing the speculum and other instruments gynecologists still use today. Sims came up with a successful surgery for fistula, a painful condition usually caused by obstructed labor that can leave women without bladder control. Historians say the procedure "revolutionized"[42] the field of modern gynecology. Sims also performed the first successful gallbladder surgery and the first successful artificial insemination.[43]

But on whom did Sims test his surgeries and tools? Who were the "guinea pigs"?[44] Enslaved Black women. Dr. Vanessa Northington Gamble, a physician and medical historian at George Washington University, explained in a special NPR series that in the 1840s, Sims spent years experimenting on enslaved women to develop a treatment for fistulas.[45] Although Sims conducted surgeries on a number of enslaved women, only the names of three are known: Anarcha, Lucy, and Betsey.

For a long time, Sims's fistula surgeries were unsuccessful. It took him four years of experimenting and a total of thirty operations on Anarcha to "perfect"[46] his method. At the time, she was a seventeen-year-old slave suffering from a fistula caused by a long and traumatic labor.

"These women were property," Dr. Gamble said. "These women could not consent. These women also had value to the slaveholders for production and reproduction—how much work they could do in the field, how many enslaved children they could produce. And by having these fistulas, they could not continue with childbirth and also have difficulty working."[47]

In his autobiography, *The Story of My Life*, Sims talks about how he negotiated with slave owners:

> I made this proposition to the owners of the negroes: If you will give me Anarcha and Betsey for experiment, I agree to perform no experiment or operation on either of them to endanger their lives, and will not charge a cent for keeping them, but you must pay their taxes and clothe them.[48]

Sims also describes how he got more slaves to test on, in addition to Anarcha, Betsey, and Lucy:

> I got three or four more to experiment on, and there was never a time that I could not, at any day, have had a subject for operation. But my operations all failed . . . this went on, not for one year, but for two and three, and even four years.[49]

Dr. Gamble points out that the surgeries, which Sims repeated again and again on the same women, including thirty times on Anarcha, were extremely painful. Sims even wrote in his biography of the results of one "stupid thing"[50] he tested that "Lucy's agony was extreme. She was much prostrated, and I thought that she was going to die. . . . After she had recovered entirely from the effects of this unfortunate experiment, I put her on a table, to examine."[51]

Although historians agree that Sims would experiment on Black women without using anesthesia and then later do the same procedures on white women *with* anesthesia, Sims himself had his own explanation. He once said that the surgeries he was perform-ing did not need anesthesia because "they are not painful enough to justify the trouble and risk."[52]

However, he also described the experimental surgeries on his enslaved subjects as "so painful, that none but a woman could have borne them."[53] But then in his autobiography, Sims writes about conducting fistula operations in Europe on wealthy women who were sedated.

Unfortunately, modern medicine has still not been able to wash away Sims's legacy. Several studies confirm that Black people con-tinue to be prescribed less pain medication.[54] As I discussed in a previous chapter, a 2016 University of Virginia study found that some doctors still believed that Black people have thicker skin and are less apt to feel pain.

In April 2018, New York City's Public Design Commission voted unanimously to remove a statue of J. Marion Sims from Cen-tral Park, following a string of protests demanding the removal of Confederate Army generals after the white supremacist protest in Charlottesville, Virginia, in 2017. The original plaque on the statue memorialized Sims for his "brilliant achievement."[55] But now, on the empty pedestal in Central Park a new plaque bears the names of Lucy, Anarcha, and Betsey, the three known women whose bodies were used by Sims without their consent.[56]

The depth of mistrust between people of color and the medical world goes much deeper than the removal of statues. We saw another example of the painful history between the medical world and African Americans when the COVID vaccine was approved toward the end of 2020. One study by Kaiser Permanente in December found that one in three Black people are hesitant about taking the COVID vaccine, making them one of the main groups most reluctant to vaccinate, along with Republicans, rural residents, and people in their thirties and forties.[57]

Why are Black people so apprehensive about the vaccine? As someone who thinks, reads, studies, and talks a lot about race, I was shocked to find the horrifying answer to that—the Tuskegee syphilis study.

This study took place between 1932 and 1972 in Alabama and was officially known as the "Tuskegee Study of Untreated Syphilis in the Negro Male."[58] The forty-year experiment was run by Public Health Service officials and studied six hundred rural Black men with syphilis over the course of their lives—the men were told they would be treated, but they were not.[59]

Although the whistleblowers brought an end to the study in 1972, the lives of those Black men and many of their families were destroyed. Scores of the men died from complications of the disease, and many of their wives and children also contracted syphilis.[60]

Researchers believe the trauma of the study still impacts African Americans to this day. The coronavirus immunization campaign is off to a shaky start in Tuskegee and other parts of Macon County. Local leaders point to a reluctance among residents because of a distrust of government promises and decades of failed health programs. Many people in this city of 8,500 also have relatives who were subjected to unethical government experimentation during the syphilis study.[61]

"It does have an impact on decisions. Being in this community, growing up in this community, I would be very untruthful if I didn't say that," Frank Lee, an emergency management director in Macon County, who is Black, told Reuters.[62]

In the 1990s, a lawsuit filed on behalf of the men by Black Tuskegee attorney Fred Gray resulted in a $9 million settlement. Then president Bill Clinton also formally apologized on behalf of the US government in 1997.[63]

But experts say the damage of the study left a legacy of distrust that is rearing its head again in the COVID fight. A December 2020 survey showed 40 percent of Black people nationwide said they wouldn't get the coronavirus vaccine. This is much higher than skepticism levels among white people, even though Black Americans have been hit disproportionately hard by the virus.[64]

I was reminded of how fresh the Tuskegee wounds remain for so many people when I read the story of Dr. Kimberly Manning in an essay for *The Lancet* medical journal called "More Than Medical Mistrust."[65]

Dr. Manning writes about her experience as a "50-year-old Black American woman physician who is a descendant of slaves"[66] volunteering to participate in a phase 3 clinical trial for a COVID vaccine in November 2020. She tells the story of how far back the connection between Tuskegee University and her family goes. Her maternal grandparents were students there. All four of their children, including Dr. Manning's mother, were born and raised in the very same hospital that conducted the untreated syphilis trials in Black men.[67]

In the following passage from her essay, Dr. Manning describes hearing the voices of her ancestors, who had no say in being tested on, as she walked up to take part in the COVID vaccine trials:

Without warning, a cacophony of sounds clattered inside of my head. Throaty voices cried out in protest. There was the tinkling of metal instruments punctuated by shrieks of pain and conciliatory murmurs. Then came scuffling sounds along with the clink of handcuffs. Someone wept in rhythmic tics and then, just for a few moments, there was silence. Next, there was the sound of a brass band playing. Then came the laughter. Soft at first, but quickly becoming louder, blended with applause and sounds of celebration. I closed my eyes and took in a deep breath, hoping I could drown it all out. I could not. . . . I sifted through my brain for more, hoping to cover not only my own queries but all of those important things that those before me had not been afforded the chance to explore. I asked and asked and asked until I ran out of questions and breath. I wish it felt like enough. It did not.[68]

Dr. Manning's words reflect the depth of the trauma that still plagues Black Americans. She says that acknowledging every aspect of the multigenerational barriers for Black Americans to enroll in clinical trials is critical to moving forward. "We are not simply untrusting—we remember," she said.[69]

History matters. Events that happened decades ago still haunt the present for many Americans. Dr. Manning is describing her struggle as a physician who knew how important a vaccine against COVID would be but also as an African American who has a "historical reluctance"[70] to assist with scientific research. And justifiably so.

But she ends her article on a hopeful note, stating that moving forward will require a collective effort. "We need a seismic shift in our relationships with Black lives, as demonstrated through government and societal actions, policies, investments, and outcomes," Dr. Manning wrote. "Medical mistrust is just the tip of a 400-year-old iceberg that has to be chipped away from every direction."[71]

Medical mistrust may indeed be the tip, but in the early summer of 2020, as COVID continued to bring the world's richest democracy to its knees, Americans were forced to face another part of this four-hundred-year-old iceberg: police brutality.

When video footage of the murder of George Floyd surfaced, it shocked Americans into a racial reckoning unlike anything we had seen before. Even former president Obama, who is usually silent on issues of activism, was moved to speak out on the killing, acknowledging during his address on Floyd's death that "we have seen in the last several weeks, the last few months, the kinds of epic changes and events in our country that are as profound as anything that I've seen in my lifetime."[72]

As most Americans remained indoors and under tight lockdown, we were forced to watch the shocking footage of an unarmed man die under the knee of a police officer. Floyd repeatedly begged the officer to let him breathe and twice called out for his mother. "Momma!" Floyd called out with his last breaths. "Momma! I'm through."[73]

Perhaps it was the isolation and toll of the pandemic, but the response from Americans to the killing was so strong and immediate, it truly felt that the country might be at a real turning point on race relations.

Even the poll numbers showed that non-Black Americans (read: white people) were finally seeing what Black Americans had been saying for decades: police brutality kills Black people. Racism is systemic in America.[74]

A Monmouth University poll taken a few days after Floyd's

death found that 71 percent of white respondents deemed racism and discrimination "a big problem"[75] in the United States, an increase of twenty-six points from 2015. Nearly 80 percent of Americans, and 75 percent of white Americans, told pollsters that the protesters' anger was either "fully" or "partially" justified.[76] Forty-nine percent of white respondents said police are more likely to use excessive force against a Black culprit than a white one, nearly double the 25 percent who acknowledged that fact in 2016.[77]

"People finally see it," Floyd's younger brother Philonise told Pulitzer Prize–winning journalist Wes Lowery in an article for *The Atlantic*. "White people, too. My brother is going to change the world."[78]

And for a moment, it really felt like that. An estimated fifteen to twenty-six million Americans of all races took to the streets to protest police brutality in the summer of 2020 in what experts say was the largest protest movement in American history.[79] The ripple effects started showing up across sectors, including corporate America. The NFL admitted they were wrong to ban players from peacefully protesting against racism. Major brands acknowledged they weren't doing enough for "diversity," some publicly announcing their support for the Black Lives Matter movement.[80]

In Minneapolis, we saw the ban of chokeholds and the charges against the officer who killed Floyd, and the three other officers involved, upgraded. In Dallas, Texas, a "duty to intervene"[81] rule was adopted, requiring officers to stop other cops who are engaging in inappropriate use of force. In New Jersey, the state announced an update to its use-of-force guidelines for the first time in decades. In Los Angeles, a motion to reduce LAPD's $1.8 billion operating budget was introduced. It went on and on.[82]

It was truly glorious to see. As a Bangladeshi, I had always been fascinated by race in America. As a little girl in the mid-1980s, I was glued to two American TV shows: *Roots* and *North and South*. Both were about slavery. Until I came to the United States for college in 1998, my knowledge of slavery in America was based on these two TV shows.

But even then, with my very limited knowledge of race, I knew that no other person of color could fathom what being Black in America was like. Even before I had the vocabulary to explain it, I knew Black in America was the hardest color to be.

In the summer of 2020, the country seemed to be falling apart, but I believed it was coming together around race. Finally. In my upper northwest DC neighborhood, people joined the protests, and all the houses put BLM signs in their yards. In the middle of a pandemic that literally isolated us, I never felt closer to my fellow Americans.

I decided to invite the author and political pundit Sophia A. Nelson, a good friend, on my podcast *Spilling Chai* for an in-depth conversation on race in America. Nelson had written an article for the *Daily Beast* entitled "Here's How We Seize the Moment George Floyd's Murder Has Created," and I wanted her to talk about this passage:

> The American people have risen. They have met the call of this moment. Something has shifted in our cities, in our suburbs, in our churches, in our culture, in our corporations, and in our hearts. And it has shifted big. America and Americans are seemingly awake from a Rip Van Winkle–like slumber as Confederate statues that never should have been erected after the Civil War and during Jim Crow are now being torn down. Unfair laws that have

given police unfettered powers to restrain and use lethal force against citizens are being revoked and rewritten. Civil rights organizations, attorneys, and a new generation of black leaders long considered unnecessary in a "post-racial" America are now very relevant again. And for the first time in my life, I am seeing and hearing people, white people, have hard, courageous, uncomfortable conversations.[83]

Nelson hits the nail on the head when she notes that after Floyd's murder, she began seeing white people have "the hard yet brave conversations"[84] around race. This is an important point because dismantling racism starts with talking about it, acknowledging it exists.

As a woman of color living in America for two decades, I thought this was huge progress, because it really is hard to talk about race with (most) white people. It's not an issue they like to acknowledge. For many, it brings up an uncomfortable history that makes them feel guilty. Many white Americans feel like they need to apologize for racism, or examine the privilege the status quo affords them. In my experience, I have found most white Americans would rather not do any of these things.

In the aftermath of George Floyd's death, though, white people suddenly seemed more willing to have "hard, courageous, uncomfortable conversations" about race.

Of course, people of color and Black people don't have the luxury of debating racism. We know it intimately. As George Floyd's death and those of many others remind us, racism literally kills. In November 2020, the American Medical Association publicly recognized that racism is a threat to public health.

I thought after the summer of 2020, we would make leaps and bounds toward racial justice because of Floyd's death, and the global momentum it gave the BLM movement would make everyone admit that, yes, racism is a problem in America. It is undeniable. It kills. It is systemic. It's in the police system, the justice system. It is in our healthcare system. And all of these are connected.

What links Floyd's death, racial justice, and the birth justice movement? What is birth justice? I asked Monica McLemore those exact questions.

"For me, I appreciate the definition of birth justice from my colleagues and collaborators, Black Women Birthing Justice, who defines birth justice as: 'We believe that birth justice exists when women and trans-folks *can* bring forward their power during pregnancy, labor, childbirth, and postpartum to make healthy decisions for themselves and their babies.'"[85]

McLemore explained to me that birth justice is part of a wider movement against reproductive oppression. It aims to dismantle inequalities of race, class, gender, and sexuality that lead to negative birth experiences, especially for women of color, low-income women, survivors of violence, immigrants, women, queer and trans folks, and women in the Global South.

"Working for birth justice involves educating the community, and challenging abuses by medical personnel and overuse of medical interventions," McLemore said. "It also involves advocating for universal access to culturally appropriate, woman-centered healthcare. It includes the right to choose whether or not to carry a pregnancy, to choose when, where, how, and with whom to birth, including access to traditional and indigenous birth-workers, such as midwives and doulas, and the right to breastfeeding support."[86]

McLemore told me she is "guided by reproductive justice and

birth justice, so the easiest way for me to describe what it means to me is that we distribute resources based on need, so that folks can have the support they need to optimize their lives including attaining whatever reproductive goals and experience they deem necessary to their existence."[87]

The prejudice and violence that exists between law enforcement and African Americans corresponds to that following women of color, especially Black women, into hospitals and delivery rooms across the country. Black women have long suffered from harmful and dangerous medical practices, as seen in America's maternal mortality deaths.

In Serena Williams's birth story, we see that women's pain is routinely dismissed even despite celebrity or the simple ability to afford quality care. In Amber Isaac's story, we see how patent disregard for her desired medical care killed her. We see how an unnecessary medical intervention, such as a C-section, cost Sha-Asia Washington her life.

"America has the worst maternal-health problems in the developed world, and there's no way to understand this without putting racism front and center," Dr. Neel Shah, an assistant professor of obstetrics, gynecology, and reproductive biology at Harvard Medical School, told the *New York Times*.[88]

In the summer of 2020, leading reproductive justice and childbirth advocacy organizations working for birth justice decided to take action. They seized the moment of George Floyd's death to have painful but necessary conversations about race to make the changes needed to save women's lives.

In a full-page ad that Every Mother Counts (EMC) had published in the *New York Times*, a national coalition came together and identified concrete actions to combat racism in maternal health settings and protect childbearing people. An open letter presented a moral question to America: "How Many Black, Brown, and Indigenous People Have to Die Giving Birth?"[89]

The letter calls for "accountability, birth justice, and legal guarantees for safe, respectful, anti-racist care."[90] The contributors are among some of the most important voices and leaders in the reproductive justice movement, such as Loretta Ross, Lynn Roberts, Angela D. Aina, Joia Crear-Perry, Dr. Jamila Taylor, along with midwife Jennie Joseph, nurse Monica R. McLemore, and doulas such as Chanel Porchia-Albert and Christine Miller, alongside the signatures of many others.[91]

These leaders came together to lay out their vision in clear steps we can take toward change, to save childbearing people's lives, and to say, "Now is the time to demand systemic change that puts Black, Brown and Indigenous communities first."[92]

The opening lines of the letter clearly declare that "racism, not race, is killing Black, Brown, and Indigenous people in our maternity care system."[93] It points to the statistic that in the United States, women are more likely to die from complications of pregnancy and birth than in fifty-four other high-resource countries, and most of these deaths are preventable.[94]

> For the first time, a woman is twice as likely to die from pregnancy-related complications as her mother was a generation ago. This burden is not equally shared. For Black, Brown, and Indigenous people, childbirth in the US is often not the joyous experience that we all deserve. Black and Indigenous women are two to three times more likely than white women to die from complications of pregnancy and birth and are also more likely to experi-

ence near misses or severe complications. One in three people of color giving birth in a hospital reports experiencing disrespectful care or mistreatment. Too often, Black, Brown, and Indigenous people are denied equal access to respectful, high-quality maternity care that is free from bias and discrimination. In maternity care units across the country, they are treated with condescension, disregard, neglect, and fear-based coercion. When asserting their rights to informed consent, bodily autonomy, and self-determination, they are subject to surveillance and policing under the same systems of structural racism that discriminate, control, and criminalize.[95]

This letter states that for Black, Brown, and Indigenous communities, birth equity is intertwined with state-sanctioned violence and police brutality. "These injustices that start at birth took the lives of Tamir Rice, Trayvon Martin, Michael Brown, Sandra Bland, George Floyd, Shantel Davis, Tony McDade, Nina Pop, Breonna Taylor, as well as Erica Garner, Shalon Irving, Kira Johnson, Amber Rose Isaac, Sha-Asia Washington, and too many other Black people who were victims of medical racism in the maternal health care system," it read.[96] "That's why birth justice matters."[97] The letter calls for action that must be rooted in reproductive justice:

Quality, equitable, and respectful care in childbirth is an essential human right. It's not enough to just talk about health equity. This is not just about implicit bias or the racism of individual providers. We need a complete systematic overhaul of the full spectrum of reproductive health care and maternity care within the US. Our hospitals, health care systems, and health insurance companies must be accountable to the people and communities they serve, center patients as experts in their care, and honor patients' rights to make decisions about their own bodies.[98]

The leaders who signed the letter state that they "envision a reality where the human rights of all people to decide whether to have or not have children and to parent children in safe and sustainable communities are protected, respected, and fulfilled, regardless of where they live or their health insurance coverage, for midwives, doulas, and perinatal support services to be fully integrated into maternity care, and for health care professions to reflect the diversity of the patients they serve."[99]

The letter also clearly lays out legislative action to take, such as passing the Black Maternal Health Momnibus Act (H.R. 6142/S.3424) in Congress, and advancing legislative proposals, like the BREATHE Act, which I take up in the next chapter.

At the end, the contributors sign off, "as leaders, organizations, and allies in the birth and reproductive justice movements, we call for institutional and governmental accountability for birth justice and legal guarantees for safe, respectful, anti-racist care, starting today. Now is the time to show to the world that birth justice matters."[100]

This letter is so important because it brings together the voices and the visions of so many people, from all walks of life, to advocate that people of color should come together to say "enough." In the midst of the hard topics such as race and police brutality and the COVID pandemic, childbearing people are demanding a complete systematic overhaul of reproductive health care and maternity care within America.

The objectives laid out in the letter may seem big and lofty to most, but they present the most actionable steps we can take. But before we can take these steps, we must acknowledge the painful history underlying such a plea and be willing to discuss it. At the very least, we need to educate ourselves about it. What some Americans think is in the past is very much in the present for African Americans and people of color.

Ibram X. Kendi is an award-winning author and founding director of the Antiracist Research and Policy Center at American University. He is considered to be one of America's foremost historians and leading anti-racist scholars. In his bestselling book *How to Be an Anti-Racist*, Kendi said that it is not enough to be "not racist."[101] He argued that the phrase has little meaning since even white nationalists such as David Duke, the former grand wizard of the Ku Klux Klan, also claim to be "not racist."

"What's the problem with being 'not racist?'" Kendi asked. "It is a claim that signifies neutrality: 'I am not a racist, but neither am I aggressively against racism.'" He said that "one either allows racial inequities to persevere, as a racist, or confronts racial inequities, as an anti-racist."[102]

Kendi wrote that for those who believe in equal opportunity and racial justice, the goal should be "anti-racist."[103] That requires persistent self-awareness, constant self-criticism, and regular self-examination. While Kendi acknowledged that being anti-racist is as essential as it is difficult, he pointed out that "the only way to undo racism is to consistently identify and describe it—and then dismantle it."[104]

Yet how can we begin to identify and describe racism if we cannot even bring ourselves to talk about it? In so many ways, people of color in America don't get to decide what's racist. White people do. I think that is a big problem, and a barrier to having hard conversations.

I have experienced this with some of my oldest and closest friends, especially during the Trump administration. I would say something he did was racist, which happened fairly often, given his appeals to the white nationalist community. Often I would find that my white friends would disagree, or suggest I use another word because calling someone racist is a bit "harsh" and incredibly "offensive."

For example, when Trump first suggested the Muslim ban, I was quick to call it racist, but my friends did not agree, or said Trump wasn't being serious about the policy. Even if the latter were true (which I'd argue it wasn't), how can we make any racial progress if we make it so hard to even talk about race?

Americans of all races need to admit that the issues of the past are very much present for so many people of color in this country. But I want to take things a step further and propose something radical: believe women of color. In recent years, we have seen how people—men and women—have a big problem believing women. They don't believe women when we say we have been raped. They don't believe women when we say we have been sexually harassed. And as I laid out in chapter 4, women are not believed when we say we are in pain. Women are not believed about our bodies. Period.

At its core, the Me Too movement asks that we *believe* women. This radical notion demands that we make believing women the default. What a revolutionary thought. Yet, we saw when Dr. Christine Blasey Ford testified on Capitol Hill against the then Supreme Court justice nominee, Brett Kavanaugh, how she was viciously attacked in the American press. What inspired such vitriol? Simple: they didn't believe her.

No matter what evidence or testimony she gave, she had no

credibility based on the fact that she was a woman. It was enough for her to be immediately disqualified in the court of public opinion. And let us not forget that Ford was an educated, privileged white woman. But that still wasn't enough for the American public.

I must reiterate: when something is bad for white women, it is worse for women of color, and the worst for Black women. My radical proposal is that we not only believe women, but we believe women of color. Believe us when we call out racism. Believe us when we say we are in pain. Hear us and believe us.

I keep coming back to the feminist author Jaclyn Friedman's essay "Deadly Silence: What Happens When We Don't Believe Women," part of the anthology *Believe Me: How Trusting Women Can Change the World* that she edited with Jessica Valenti. Friedman calls not believing women a public health crisis, a very important point of hers that I cite in chapter 3. She goes on to say that women's believability is worse than it looks.

Friedman says women are subjected to a double whammy: women are held to much higher standards than men before they are believed, and people actually prefer not to find women credible. "As a culture, we hate to believe women, and we penalize them for forcing us to do so," Friedman wrote.[105]

She says as the credibility of women increases, especially when it goes against gender norms, their likability in society decreases. "They become shrill bitches, ball busters, too aggressive, too bossy, such intolerable know-it-alls," Friedman said. "It is not enough that we demand women clear a much higher bar than men do to prove their trustworthiness. It's that we're mad when they manage to succeed anyway. And we're all paying the price for that anger."[106]

Friedman makes a crucial point when she recognizes that the systemic disbelief of women has less to do with actually seeing women as untrustworthy, and more about being afraid of what happens if women are able to step into our full power. She points out that this distinction doesn't matter in practice.[107]

Friedman asked if antiabortion activists "really think women are so easily duped by doctors, or is it just more convenient for them to blame 'doctors' and posit women as frail-minded and in need of protection than it is to admit that they just want to dictate what we do with our own bodies? Do we not believe that trans women know themselves better than we do, or do we just fear how destabilizing it is to admit that gender is a construct? The damage is done either way."[108]

Friedman wrote that because the existing power structure is built on female subjugation, female credibility is innately dangerous to it. She explained this further in the following passage:

Patriarchy is called that for a reason: men really do benefit from it. When we take seriously women's experiences of sexual violence and humiliation, men will be forced to lose a kind of freedom they often don't even know they enjoy: the freedom to use women's bodies to shore up their egos, convince themselves they are powerful and in control, or whatever other uses they see fit. When we genuinely believe in women's leadership capacity, men must face twice the competition they previously had to contend with. And none of us, whatever our gender, are immune from the tremors that can come when the assumptions at the foundation of our social contracts are upended.[109]

I think Friedman makes such an important point by stating that believing women can ultimately dismantle the patriarchy by making women credible. Why would men allow that to happen when they benefit so much from the existing power structure? Believing women is a danger to their power.

Furthermore, viewing women as "fully human"[110] may come at the price of taking away certain kinds of oppressive power from men, but the rest of the human race would benefit hugely. "It should be enough to believe in women simply because it's better for women," Friedman wrote. "But for every time it isn't, remember this: the costs of disbelieving us are astronomical, and no one escapes the bill."[111]

And therein lies a crucial message—believing women, investing in our health and rights, does not just benefit us. It benefits all of humanity. And when we deny women credibility, the price is huge. As Friedman said, no one escapes the bill. Men and women pay.[111]

During the midst of this pandemic, we have been exposed to so many parallel pandemics, many of which have existed longer than COVID: the pandemic of racism, police brutality, maternal health, and the "shadow pandemic" of domestic violence.

But I really think COVID is giving us a huge opportunity by showing us all these devastating crises. They are not unsolvable. Justice is possible and so within our reach. We have a real chance now to take steps toward justice—in race relations and maternal health. We can start by listening to women—and to insist on support for our choices about how, and when, we give birth.

What a radical idea. Imagine what would happen if we believed women, if we listened to women of color.

The following and final chapters present a few scenarios and solid, actionable plans to do just that.

8

How to Be Your Own
Best Health Advocate

It was 1999, I was a sophomore at the University of Virginia, and I had just heard Gloria Steinem speak on campus a month ago. Having fully embraced the "feminist" label, which was still considered "controversial" at the time, I started a feminist club called the International Women's Organization (IWO). This group of fifteen to twenty fellow students of color gathered monthly at the coffee shop in Alderman Library. We talked about global women's rights issues and about what feminism meant to us.

Even though IWO had no real impact on the larger fight for women's rights, I am proud of myself for creating a space for people of color and diverse perspectives at a predominantly white college. And I did it. It was also a space where we celebrated strong voices of color instead of just viewing Black and Brown women as "affirmative action" cases.

In a similar vein, this chapter ends on a hopeful note. As I wrap up my discussion of depression, domestic violence, preventable deaths in childbirth, and COVID, I contend that this is not a "doom and gloom" book. The issues I raise here shouldn't make us feel helpless. On the contrary, they should motivate us to make a difference and play our part.

So many of the challenges I examine in this book are solvable and preventable. We are not dealing with cancer or AIDS, where so much still depends on unknowns. It is within our power to stand up for women. We can and should intervene and speak up to save women's lives.

In this chapter, I profile courageous women of color—activists who are dedicated to saving women's lives and campaigning for the compensation we are due. If the pandemic is showing us anything, it is how much we need and rely upon the labor of women, but how we almost never pay them—in respect or money. Therefore, I have included a cross section of solutions women are putting out in the world. As dark as it may seem, the pandemic presents us with an unprecedented opportunity to get right what we have gotten wrong for too long.

This chapter profiles the work and initiatives of twenty-first-century pioneers in women's health—women such as Girls Who Code founder Reshma Saujani and her new plan for moms crippled by the pandemic; pioneering midwife Jennie Joseph and her compassionate-care model that consistently results in healthy mothers and babies; women's health policy expert Dr. Jamila Taylor; and Every Mother Counts managing director of policy, advocacy, and grantmaking, Nan Strauss.

Although I firmly reiterate that the onus should not be on women to be believed, the chapter also includes a "tool kit" of questions to ask, research to do, and ways to advocate for yourself as a woman of color that may help you avoid becoming another statistic.

Reshma Saujani, the Marshall Plan for Moms

Many of us know Reshma Saujani from Girls Who Code, the international nonprofit organization whose aim is to close the gender gap in technology. Saujani began her career as an attorney and activist. In 2010, she burst onto the political scene as the first Indian American woman to run for US Congress (D-NY).[1]

She is also the author of the international bestseller *Brave, Not Perfect* and the *New York Times* bestseller *Girls Who Code: Learn to Code and Change the World*. Saujani's TED Talk, "Teach Girls Bravery, Not Perfection" has more than five million views, and she is also the host of the award-winning podcast *Brave, Not Perfect*.[2]

While Saujani is no stranger to disrupting the game, as COVID ravaged and unraveled the lives of women across America, she was spurred to action. Her organization took out a full-page ad in *The New York Times* as a letter addressed to President Biden proposing the "Marshall Plan for Moms."[3]

"This pandemic has shown us just how little we value motherhood—and that is to say, we do not value motherhood at all," Saujani said.[4] "We have been fighting for women's equality for centuries. We are at a moment to finish that fight and rebuild our economy to finally value women's work. And not only that, but send a signal to girls that women's labor counts; that their careers, their dreams won't be taken for granted."[5]

The Marshall Plan for Moms says motherhood is a job and women must be paid. COVID has made that clear. The plan was signed by fifty high-profile women activists and creatives, including the leaders of the Women's March and the Me Too movement, and Hollywood actresses.[6]

"We are in a national crisis that is affecting mothers," Saujani explained to me.[7] "There are three working moms unemployed for every one dad. And so we wanted to bring together a coalition of women—including Julianne Moore, Gabrielle Union, Amy Schumer, Whitney Wolfe Herd, Jennifer Hyman, Eva Longoria, and others to call on the Biden administration to put together a Marshall Plan for Moms to get moms back to work. This plan would include means-tested basic income to women, paid leave, affordable day care, pay equity. Beyond that, we need a plan to get schools to reopen for 5 days a week, and for Wall Street and Main Street to step up and think about how we're retraining and hiring moms who've been forced to leave the workforce. And all of this can't just be a stopgap for the rest of the year, it needs to live on past this pandemic."

Modeled after the 1948 Marshall Plan, a US government initiative that provided financial investments to rebuild Europe after World War II, the plan urges the government to pay mothers a $2,400 monthly stipend for their labor throughout the COVID-19 pandemic. It also calls for paid family leave, affordable childcare, and pay equity.[8]

"Since March, our mothers have been working simultaneously as teachers and counselors and cleaners and nurses and nannies and chefs and tech support and the list goes on and on and on," Saujani wrote in *The Hill* in December 2020. "Countless millions of women have been forced to cut their working hours, scale back their careers, or leave the workforce entirely in order to be full-time caregivers. It's true that not all caregivers are women, but the vast majority are."[9]

Saujani tells the government exactly what is needed and what to do. The letter reads:

Dear President Biden:

You know this well: moms are the bedrock of society. And we're tired of working for free.

We need a Marshall Plan for Moms—Now.

Like the original Marshall Plan of 1948, this plan would be a financial investment in rebuilding from the ground up.

COVID has decimated so many of our careers. Two million of us have left the workforce, at a rate of four times that of men in September alone. Millions more have been forced to cut back our hours or work around the clock to keep our jobs and be full-time caregivers.

This is not an isolated incident—it is a national crisis. You didn't create this problem, but your administration has an opportunity to fix it.[10]

The letter asks the government to:

- Establish a task force to create a Marshall Plan for Moms.
- Implement a short-term monthly payment to moms depending on needs and resources.
- Pass long-overdue policies like paid family leave, affordable childcare, and pay equity.

Finally, the letter demands that "it's time to put a dollar figure on our labor. Motherhood isn't a favor and it's not a luxury. It's a job."[11]

Saujani knows what she is talking about and she knows what moms need because she's one of us. "I've been living this since March," Saujani said in an interview with *Forbes*. "When Covid happened, I became my son's Kindergarten teacher while supposedly being on maternity leave for my other child and being a CEO of a very large organization. I was seeing the pain and exhaustion I was feeling on my Zoom screen with the women that worked for me, and the women that I was working with. The breaking point for me was when schools closed again in New York City. When most public school districts decided to do hybrid learning, they didn't ask mothers if we would take this on. They just assumed that we would do it. You realize how little they value our labor."[12]

Saujani is not proposing her plan as a magic wand that will fix all of women's problems. "To be clear, a Marshall Plan for Moms will not solve the deeply rooted norms that make women our default caregivers in the first place," Saujani wrote in *The Hill*. "The battle against those norms—against our hugely damaging structural inequities—doesn't end with a monthly stipend from the federal government. What might end, or at least begin to abate, is the gross disregard for the value of mothers' unpaid, unseen, unappreciated labor."

Saujani points out that this plan will not only give women the support they need until they can go back to work, it will also stimulate the economy, and send an important message to little girls and young women across America: "that our society values the contributions of women, and that their careers, dreams, and lives will not be taken for granted."

During a pandemic that has expected so much of mothers, wouldn't that be a great message to hear?

"We, in nine months, lost 30 years of progress," said Saujani to

CBS News in February 2021. "Think about that. The reality is, is we are in a moment of rage. Every mother I know has just had it."[13]

Jennie Joseph, Commonsense Childbirth

Jennie Joseph is a British-trained midwife who is the CEO and founder of Commonsense Childbirth, a nonprofit she founded in 1998. It operates a midwifery school and perinatal professional training institute, health clinics, and a birthing center in Orlando, Florida.

Jennie created the JJ Way, an evidence-based maternal health model delivering readily accessible, patient-centered, culturally congruent care to women in areas that she calls "materno-toxic zones." It is a "patient-centered model of care."[14]

A growing body of research links stress, racism, and maternal health issues. Jennie believes that those factors also contribute to high rates of maternal illness among African American women. "The daily assault that you deal with, just being of color, it's so lethal," she said to the *New York Times*. "The stress, the judgment, it's killing our babies."[15]

According to their website, the JJ Way model "is effective in reducing disparities and improving outcomes because it operates from the premise that every woman wants a healthy baby and that every woman deserves one."[16] It also encourages patients and their family supporters to "operate the same way and are therefore invited in as an integral part of each prenatal visit."[17] The JJ Way's key components in their healthcare delivery are:

- Prenatal bonding through respect, support, education, encouragement, and empowerment.

- Freedom of choice: labor and delivery can take place in any location the woman feels most comfortable.
- Take the fear of unmedicated or out-of-hospital childbirth out of the equation.
- Work with our physician partners to ensure a smooth transition of care for women who prefer to birth at the hospital.

But what makes the JJ Way different from other prenatal care? Firstly, Jennie accepts anyone as a patient regardless of ability to pay or health insurance status, she tells the *New York Times*.[18] Second, Jennie considers her staff—the receptionists, medical assistants, and educators—not as her assistants or the people who get the patient ready to see the provider, but "as critical parts of the team that help mothers get to term safely."[19]

Jennie emphasizes that the time her clients spend with her staff is almost more important than the time spent with her or another provider in her practice. And lastly, she goes to great lengths to ensure that she and her staff treat patients with respect and consideration.

One of the first principles of Jennie's model is offering *access*. And it's not just about helping women who can't pay. She also helps women with pregnancies that other clinics deem "too high-risk"[20] to deal with. Jennie won't turn away anyone on the basis of how far along her pregnancy is. "We regularly deal with tears at the front door," she said in an interview with the *Times*. She says patients regularly say to her, "I can't believe you're actually going to help me."[21]

The JJ Way sounds so simple, but what are the results? For the roughly six hundred women Jennie sees annually, they have been impressive. The *Times* reports that recent outside evaluation of her work, funded by the West Orange Healthcare District, found significantly lower rates of preterm birth and low infant birth weight among her patients than in other settings. Joseph's clients of African descent were almost 40 percent less likely than women of a similar race throughout the nation to have a preterm labor or a child with a low birth weight.[22]

Jennie and I met through Christy at SXSW and became instant friends. But Jennie's welcome to America was not nearly as warm. When she first arrived in Florida in the 1980s, she was just thirty years old. Within a year, she was happily married and working with an obstetrician. He offered to help Jennie with her endometriosis-related pain through surgery. After four unsuccessful surgeries with him that only left her with more pain, Jennie went to get a second opinion. This doctor recommended a hysterectomy, which she agreed to.

But the surgery left her without her uterus *and* her ovaries. Jennie was devastated, because she did not realize that most women who undergo hysterectomies keep their ovaries, allowing them to have more children through a surrogate if they choose to. Her husband was furious, and she felt powerless. While she acknowledges she did not ask the right questions, the experience woke her up to the reality of being a Black woman in America. She was grateful for the one child she already had, but the option of having more was gone. The horrific experience woke Jennie up and lit a fire in her to stand up for all women through the "vehicle of midwifery."[23]

Jennie feels strongly about how women are treated in a system where "we don't know what to ask, we haven't got a voice, we are not heard," she said in an interview with NBC News. This is especially true for Black women, Indigenous women, any woman that is considered "other."[24]

Jennie points out that the JJ Way is a simple, cost-effective model that can be "easily emulated and adapted for any practice." That outlook made Jennie all the more ready to treat women when the pandemic hit. In an exclusive interview, she told me that the JJ Way is going virtual: "Virtual Maternity Care—The JJ Way."[25] She says that the training program for clinicians is launching in spring 2021, and the pilot is already showing extremely promising outcomes and high patient satisfaction.

"One of the things I'm seeing for sure is that now they're [patients] settling in," Jennie said. "They're getting to that place of calming themselves back down. My patients in particular have become very comfortable with telehealth, which I didn't think would actually be the case, so we pivoted very quickly to telehealth. But not in the way that people might understand telehealth. We were able to prove that we could do telehealth and still maintain relationships."

Jennie says that telehealth has its challenges. After all, health professionals have to bond and connect with women, give them the dignity and respect they deserve while relieving their fears—all over a phone or video call, during a global pandemic.

To make her clients feel more connected to care, Jennie sends them their own fetal doppler, blood-pressure cuffs, and analysis sticks, so they can do more at-home testing and monitoring between telehealth sessions.

"These physical kits are enabling them to be empowered; they can put the doppler on their baby's heartbeat," Jennie says. "And I think that went a long way to them accepting and being comfortable with telehealth, so overarchingly what I've seen is that you can run obstetric care safely and, you know, with good outcomes. We have had amazing outcomes, you got great satisfaction scores. This is what I'm now calling 'Virtual Maternity Care—The JJ Way.' I did this whole new model."

Jennie said the pilot has been going great, and because she has the training and accreditation, it makes moving the program onto an online platform even easier. She admits if it had not been for the pandemic, she most likely wouldn't have created a new program.

"We've always been very in touch with our moms with the phone calls, check-ins, you name it," Jennie told me. "We've used video when they needed it or they've asked for it. COVID showed me that mothers who normally wouldn't be accepting of that modality are."

And Jennie says it's some of the most disenfranchised women who have in many ways experienced the most "continual assaults" on their health who are the people who have pivoted with Jennie and her team. "They are now okay with telehealth as a way to receive maternity care to stay safe," she said. Previously, she pointed out, many people were understandably hesitant about telehealth. They didn't think it was safe, they didn't feel good about it, or they didn't know if their providers were listening to them.

She brings up Amber Isaac, the young woman who died after giving birth to her son in New York in the summer of 2020. Isaac was the young woman who repeatedly tried to sound the alarm about needing to be seen in person, but she was ignored. Her falling platelet issue was never resolved. Ultimately, she died unnecessarily.

When I asked Jennie if she believed COVID was giving us an opportunity with maternal health to get on the right path to place women's needs in the center of their care, she agreed—to a point.

"It gives us this opportunity to just call it like it is, to tell the truth," Jennie said. "That's one of my hashtags. Here's what COVID did—it allowed for us to say our truth again, but this time to be heard because we've had this opportunity. I mean, we've had a racism pandemic for as long as I've been here."

Jennie acknowledges that the maternal health crisis was in "full force" when she first arrived from Britain in the 1990s. She says that the pandemic has allowed "belief and recognition and acknowledgment that [what advocates have been saying] is true." Maternal health in America is a public health emergency. Everything else up to now has been "[like] 'Oh yeah, well,'" Jennie said in terms of the public's lack of concern. She said the good thing is how COVID has brought awareness to this issue because "America needs continual awareness."

When I asked Jennie about how she thinks the pandemic is making pregnant women (particularly non-Black women) consider alternatives to out-of-hospital births, she described it as "powerful." Many folks are discovering midwifery for the first time.

But Jennie notes that despite the positives, the more things change, the more they stay the same. The surge in out-of-hospital births also makes some hospitals panic. They may not be sure how to incorporate the interest in out-of-hospital births under the scope of their business model, which for hospitals is a "capital-first" approach to maternal and child health.

Jennie makes an important point: that just because the public is more aware that they have out-of-hospital birth options doesn't necessarily translate to hospitals and birth centers collaborating for the benefit of pregnant women. Jennie says it is more than the competition stepping up. For hospitals, it is about their bottom line, and at the end of the day it means more business might be "going outside instead of staying inside."

"This is why hospitals create such pretend things such as in-hospital birth centers," Jennie said. She questions what an "in-hospital birthing center" even is.

"It's another excuse, you know," she said. "That's why they put up curtains and put panels and furnishings and say you can bring your lavender." But no matter how much they try to act like they can offer the same personalized care you get from midwifery, they can't.

For Jennie, it all comes back to listening to women. With the pandemic, we have the opportunity to fulfill what women say they need. "We've had a lot of data collection, research, et cetera," she said. "And then we just go back to where we need more. Let's just get something done. Can we listen, this time with the new approach of what's needed and then can we put it into action? Where's the policy behind the listening? Where are the changes that are not impossible to do?"

She says COVID has shown us that governments have the money. It's not a funding issue. "It's time to do the action on the listening, because when we listen we actually find out what people truly want and need," Jennie said. "And it doesn't sound like what we've got."

Dr. Jamila Taylor, the Century Foundation

Dr. Jamila Taylor is one of the most important policy experts and advocates in the maternal health space, especially when it comes to reproductive health and rights. But Jamila and I go way back to our early days of lobbying on the Hill. In those days, she was one of the few women of color in a position of influence. When I worked at the Feminist Majority, if my boss needed anything confirmed about upcoming legislation, she would have me call Jamila.

Today, Dr. Taylor is the director of health care reform and a senior fellow at the Century Foundation, where she leads the organization's work to build on the Affordable Care Act and "develop the next generation of health reform to achieve high-quality, affordable, and universal coverage in America."[26]

But she's also a global leader and recognized authority in women's health whose career has focused on reproductive rights and justice, the structural barriers to healthcare, racial and gender disparities in health outcomes, and the intersection between healthcare and economic justice.

She was previously a senior fellow and director of the women's health and rights program at the Center for American Progress, and a senior adviser at Ipas, a global NGO dedicated to ending preventable deaths and disabilities from unsafe abortions.

We have stayed friends over the last two decades, and whenever I have any questions she is still my go-to policy expert. But when I interviewed her for this book, the conversation got personal fast. Jamila told me that one of the most effective ways she has found to deal with medical racism and medical mistrust in her own life is choosing Black providers. She says it has made a big difference.

Jamila in no way suggests that using providers of color will solve all the discrimination in healthcare because "even people of color can be racist."[27]

Nevertheless, she said, "Once it clicked for me that I'm more likely to have better health outcomes, and a better experience navigating the healthcare system, both for myself and my child, I started to make a concerted effort to seek out providers of color, particularly Black providers for both myself and my kid. I'm talking about everything like specialists, primary care, dentists, and that really hit me when I was pregnant with my son. It has meant a world of difference."

Jamila says this epiphany impacts the nature of the conversations with her providers. "Because they are Black providers, they also have a sense of the unique lived experience that I may have as a mother, as a Black woman, that my son may have as a young Black boy," Jamila said. "So that has been major for me and my family. My providers listen to me, they give me advice, they're accessible."

She is aware that when she advocates for herself in this situation, it's not the same life or death issue women of color may find themselves facing within the medical system. "I know that that's a privilege," Jamila said. "I know that most people that look like me, they may not be able to have that experience. So I think that is key."

Jamila said that when her son was little, having a Black pediatrician was really key. "Even now, I always ask my friends, like, do you have a Black doctor?" she says. "You know, because it depends on what area you live in. I will say that it's been generally easier living in the DC area to be able to find providers that look like me, but it's not always like that if you're living in a rural area, or like Indiana."

She points out that it's not just about Black doctors but having perinatal support workers, nurses, and ensuring that the "pipeline of healthcare professionals" at all levels are a "diverse set of folks." Jamila says it's important we bring them into the fold "because that's a critical aspect of promoting the health of people of color."

When I ask if she's hopeful after having the pandemic blow the lid off America's women's health crisis that people will take women's health seriously, Jamila says she is.

"You and me, we were already in the space, and we knew how dire it was in the context of women's health overall, and maternal health was this bomb, you know, and then COVID came along," she explained. "COVID was the light bulb. Not just in this country, but even internationally, folks are looking at the US, and it clicks for people. 'Oh, this is what they mean when they talk about systemic racism and the healthcare system.'"

Jamila points to how Black and Hispanic people are more likely to get critically ill from COVID and die from it. She said the pandemic helped people to see that the disparity in healthcare outcomes across the board is real, not just something that people working in the health equity space have been harping on for the past four decades. "So I am encouraged," Jamila said.

She notes that the CDC's preliminary data shows that Black and Hispanic pregnant women who get COVID are more likely to get critically ill. "There's no other thing," she said. "It's touching every aspect of people's lives." But she thinks we must talk about the economic piece of COVID, too.

She points out how there are clear costs associated with COVID treatment and lost productivity, especially when millions of people don't have healthcare, or they've lost their employer-sponsored healthcare. "People are having to grapple with paid leave as an issue," Jamila continued. "So all of those things are connected, and we need to be talking about them in an intersectional way."

Perhaps the most important part of my conversation with Jamila was about how women of color feel they are expected to "fix things."

"People are always looking to us to save everything," Jamila said. "But when we need saving, there's no need to save us. You know, Stacey Abrams, save democracy in Georgia . . . There're so many examples of people of color to come in, and just expected to come and clean things up."

A literal case in point occurred after the Capitol riots of January 6, 2021. It was Black custodians who swept up the shattered glass and the mess made by white supremacist rioters. The images were jarring.

"Because I worked on the Hill for a number of years, that had already clicked for me," she recalled. "As far back as I can remember, like the custodial staff and the groundskeepers, they're predominantly Black. And think of how that must feel. That crap is unbelievable."

Nan Strauss, managing director of policy, advocacy, and grantmaking for Every Mother Counts (EMC)

Nan Strauss leads EMC's efforts to advance policies and programs that expand access to quality, respectful, and equitable care practices for all members of the community. She previously worked as the director of research and policy at Choices in Childbirth, where her work included research and advocacy on high-value models of maternity care that align with the "Triple Aim"[28] for healthcare improvement.

Strauss served as the director of maternal health research and policy with Amnesty International USA, where she worked on issues related to maternal health and the right to health. She was the lead researcher and coauthor of the groundbreaking report *Deadly Delivery: The Maternal Health Care Crisis in the USA.*

Prior to joining Amnesty, Strauss was a staff attorney at the Center for Reproductive Rights where she litigated cases in federal court. Her litigation included challenging the US Food and Drug Administration's refusal to make emergency contraception available over the counter to women of all ages.

I spoke with Nan about EMC's legislative goals and asked her if she's feeling hopeful about them with the Biden-Harris administration, especially given Vice President Harris's senatorial work on maternal health.[29]

"This administration has already shown a strong commitment to health, health equity, and maternal health, which makes us very optimistic about the opportunity for meaningful and durable changes," Nan told me. "Vice President Harris has been a committed advocate for maternal health, especially as it affects Black women. She sponsored the Maternal CARE Act, and served as the Senate sponsor of the Black Maternal Health Momnibus in 2020. There is so much momentum already in Congress."

Nan says while the pandemic has been disastrous overall, it has also generated opportunities to reenvision what maternity care can look like. "This is a chance to transform the maternity care system in ways that make meaningful, long-lasting, durable changes that will continue to improve maternal health beyond the pandemic," she told me.

She gives three examples of areas where the pandemic has highlighted opportunities that can improve America's maternal health in the long term: (1) demand for community birth and the midwifery model of care; (2) opportunities to expand telehealth to reduce the burden on pregnant people; and (3) the need for informational and systems navigation support from doulas and other perinatal support service providers (e.g., lactation support, childbirth education, peer mental health support).

When we turned our conversation to EMC's legislative goals, Nan was clear that priorities are to extend Medicaid coverage from the current two months to a full year postpartum. Nan stresses that for EMC this goal would be for all states, permanently, with a bump in federal matching funds to 100 percent.

That is followed by wanting to expand equitable access to high-value models of maternity care proven to result in positive outcomes and experiences, while also being cost-effective, such as the midwifery model of care, supporting community doulas, and establishing more birth centers. EMC's third goal is shifting the focus to respectful care and creating a system that provides transparency and holds government and health systems accountable for quality and respectful care.

Here are the relevant specific pieces of legislation that have been previously introduced in Congress that support each of these priorities:

- Black Maternal Health Momnibus Act: Led by the Black Maternal Health Caucus and sponsored by Congresswomen Lauren Underwood and Alma Adams in the House and Senator Cory Booker in the Senate, the Black Maternal Health Momnibus is a package of twelve pieces of legislation that advances inclusive and accessible maternity care, particularly addressing disparities in maternal health outcomes that disproportionately affect Black and Indigenous childbearing people. The Black Maternal Health Momnibus was first introduced in 2020 and was reintroduced in the 117th Congress in February 2021. Its policies include investing in the social determinants of health, funding community-based organizations, promoting a diverse maternity care workforce, instituting implicit bias and anti-racism training, and advancing respectful maternity care during public health emergencies.

- MOMMIES Act (S. 1343 / H.R. 2602): Sponsored by Senator Cory Booker in the Senate and Congresswoman Ayanna Pressley in the House, the MOMMIES Act aims to improve maternal health outcomes by targeting care access, quality, cost, and experience. Among other provisions, this bill will extend Medicaid coverage to a year following childbirth; pilot maternity care homes, a model that provides coordinated, comprehensive, and culturally appropriate services and care; and assess and recommend strategies to expand Medicaid coverage of doula care.

- MOMMA's Act (S. 916 / H.R. 1897): Sponsored by Senator Dick Durbin and Congresswoman Robin Kelly, the Mothers and Offspring Mortality and Morbidity Awareness (MOMMA) Act seeks to prevent maternal mortality by providing assistance to states regarding best practices in maternal mortality identification and review, increasing access to care, and expanding training in cultural competence. It extends Medicaid coverage from two months to a year following childbirth; supports the expansion of "safety bundles" to improve maternity care; and establishes Centers of Excellence for implicit bias and cultural competency education.

- Helping MOMS Act (H.R. 4996): Sponsored by Congresswoman Ayanna Pressley, Congresswoman Robin Kelly, Congresswoman Lauren

Underwood, Congressman Michael Burgess, MD, Congressman Buddy Carter, Congresswoman Jaime Herrera Beutler, and Congresswoman Cathy McMorris Rodgers, the Helping MOMS Act is bipartisan legislation aimed at reducing and ending America's growing maternal mortality crisis. The bill contains key provisions of the Healthy MOMMIES Act, which Congresswoman Pressley introduced in 2019. This bipartisan bill allows states to submit a state plan amendment to provide one year of postpartum coverage through Medicaid and the Children's Health Insurance Program. It directs the Medicaid and CHIP Payment Access Commission (MACPAC) to publish a report on doula support under Medicaid coverage and recommendations for improvement.

- Midwives for MOMS Act (H.R. 3849): This is a bipartisan bill that seeks to improve maternal health outcomes; ensure access to high-quality maternal health services for women, newborns, individuals, and families; and help end crisis-level US maternal mortality rates by expanding educational opportunities for Certified Nurse-Midwives (CNMs) and Certified Midwives (CMs). The unprecedented, monumental legislation represents the first time that federal policymakers have prioritized investment in accredited midwifery education programs. This bill establishes funding streams through the Human Resources & Services Administration to increase the number of midwives available to women, specifically midwives of color and from other underrepresented groups.

- Perinatal Workforce Act (H.R. 6164): This bill, a part of the Black Maternal Health Momnibus, is sponsored by Congresswoman Gwen Moore and addresses the "maternity care deserts" in the United States that have no hospitals offering obstetric care and zero obstetric providers. It provides guidance for states on recruiting a diverse midwifery workforce and incorporating midwives into collaborative, culturally congruent care teams, and a Government Accountability Office report on barriers to entering the midwifery workforce and recommendations for addressing such barriers.

- TRICARE for Coverage of Doula Support Act (S. 3826): This legislation would expand TRICARE coverage to include doula support, which offers continuous nonclinical one-to-one emotional, physical, and informational support before, during, and after birth. Studies have shown that doula support can improve maternal and infant outcomes while reducing costs of maternity care. It provides pregnant TRICARE beneficiaries with doulas and other maternity support services.

- BABIES Act (H.R. 5189): Another bipartisan bill, this time cosponsored by Congresswoman

Katherine Clark and Congressman Buddy Carter, it would establish a demonstration model for birth centers in six states for women in areas with limited access to care. This model of care has been shown in the Strong Start Initiative to reduce preterm and low birth weight births, reduce cesarean births, and lead to significant cost savings due to better outcomes. It establishes a Medicaid demonstration program to develop and advance innovative payment models for freestanding birth center services.

- The Kira Johnson Act (H.R. 6144): A part of the Black Maternal Health Momnibus, this bill would increase funding for community-based organizations that are leading the charge to protect moms, in addition to supporting training programs and accountability mechanisms to address bias and racism in maternity care settings. It would create the Respectful Maternity Care compliance program to establish respectful maternity care compliance offices in hospitals, health systems, and other maternity care delivery settings to institutionalize reporting on incidences of bias, racism, discrimination, and mistreatment.

- Maternal Health Pandemic Response Act (S. 4769 / H.R. 8027): Sponsored by Senator Elizabeth Warren and Congresswomen Lauren Underwood, in addition to other COVID-19 recovery efforts, this bill creates a task force on respectful maternity care practices (with measures to address and identify racism and bias in care delivery). It will translate changes made during COVID-19 pandemic response into long-term systemic change.

That's a lot of bills, which I think is fantastic news. Strauss agrees. She tells me that having so many pieces of legislation drafted and ready to go gives her hope.

"There are an unprecedented number of very strong bills in the pipeline that would improve maternal health and health equity, many with bipartisan support," she said. "We are continuing to build on past efforts to draft legislation that will advance maternal health in the US to continue our work towards respectful, quality, and equitable maternity care for all."

9

The Truth about Treatment
for Women of Color

I t is ironic that I am writing this chapter on advocating for yourself in the American healthcare system. First, I am a Bangladeshi
woman from one of the poorest countries on earth, telling American women how they can work to improve the American healthcare
system for their own benefit. It is still something I struggle with—
questioning doctors, challenging their medical expertise. It is not
how I was raised. Growing up in the eighties, your doctor's word
might as well have been the word of God. It takes a lot of courage
to push back, but when it comes to our health, we have no choice.

"Traditionally, we don't advocate for ourselves," Dr. Joi
Bradshaw-Terrell, an ob-gyn in Chicago, told NBC News.[1] "Historically, Black women have been taught to see a physician, they
tell you something, and you just do it. You don't ask questions."[2]

Feminist author Maya Dusenbery agrees and says just by being
a woman, it's already hard to stand up for yourself.

"Advocating for yourself as a woman patient can be challenging," Dusenbery told me.[3] "On the one hand, you may need to be

assertive to be taken seriously. On the other hand, you may worry that if you push too hard, you'll be seen as a difficult, demanding patient. Unfortunately, that fear is sometimes very justified. That's why it's important to remember that gender bias in medicine is a systemic problem that can't be fixed just by individual patients better advocating for themselves."

One of the easiest things women can do to better advocate for themselves is to bring someone with them to doctors' appointments whenever possible.

"Many of the women I interviewed felt that having a male partner or family member or friend corroborate the severity of their symptoms made providers take them more seriously," Maya Dusenbery told NPR in an interview about her own book in March 2018.[4] "Which is a sad testament to the sexism so many women face. But I think having any ally with you can be helpful."

"Above all, it's so important to trust that you know when something is not right with your body," Dusenbery said. "It's all too easy for even the most empowered women to start second-guessing themselves when an expert in a white coat with years of schooling is dismissing their concerns. Remember that doctors are human beings who can make mistakes, and medical knowledge is incomplete. Keep seeking another opinion until you find a healthcare provider who listens to you and is willing to say, 'I don't know what's wrong' and roll up their sleeves when faced with symptoms they can't readily explain."

I asked Gabrielle Jackson, author of *Pain and Prejudice*, what she thinks are the most effective ways women can advocate for themselves.

"This is a really difficult question, and it's complicated to give an answer to, because I don't really think that women can do all that much to be taken seriously," Jackson said. "All the suggestions people usually give to women to be taken more seriously are often signs doctors use to categorize women as either hysterical or 'highly anxious about her health,' which make them even less likely to be taken seriously."[5]

Jackson is not optimistic about the options women have. "Taking test results and a symptoms diary to an emergency room is probably the worst possible action to take—doctors will laugh you out of the emergency room, or at least send you home and then laugh behind your back. 'Doctor shopping' is actually one of the actions doctors look for in dismissing women or writing them off with some kind of functional disorder (modern terminology for 'hysterical'). If you're a woman of color, or transgender, insisting on being taken seriously could see you labeled 'aggressive' or 'difficult' or 'attention seeking' and also not likely to improve your chances of being taken seriously or having your concerns addressed. It really cannot be left up to women (again!) to change medicine."

Jackson tells me the only good advice she can honestly give is to find a general practitioner (GP) or family doctor you know and trust and build a relationship with them.

"A good GP will be your best advocate for care and your best chance of being taken seriously by other specialists," she said. "They can also help you find other doctors that are true experts in the area you need. Keep going back to this doctor and update them on all your treatment and care."

But many experts say that asking questions is the place to start. Medical misdiagnosis is the third leading cause of death in the United States, killing about 400,000 people each year.[6] Asking questions is one of the most important things we can do to save our lives.

Amy Mason-Cooley, whom we met in an earlier chapter, is a

sickle cell disease advocate whose pain was dismissed until she almost died.

"As a Black woman I would advise *all of us* to speak out," Mason-Cooley told me.

"Don't settle for mediocre care," she stressed. "Our lives are just as valuable, and it's time to make others see that. Given the history of care and the stereotype 'strong Black woman,' it is OK to have *feelings*. It's OK to admit your pain. It's OK to place that title down and make your situation known."[7]

Mason-Cooley recalled to NBC News that once she was left in a hospital waiting room for ten hours until she passed out from pain. She woke up to a nurse telling her, "This isn't a pain clinic," implying that Mason-Cooley was seeking drugs.

"I have straight-up told doctors and nurses, 'If I wanted it to get high, I could do it on the streets for cheaper, with less judgment,'" she told NBC. "I'm here because I'm sick."[8]

Mason-Cooley says that she has heard of similar issues from other people of color, especially Black people who also suffer from sickle cell disease. She says those who may experience pain in the middle of the night force themselves to wait until the morning to go to the hospital because they know a 2:00 a.m. trip to the emergency room for severe pain would only "result in accusations that they are addicts."[9]

But I asked Mason-Cooley how women of color, especially Black women, can advocate for themselves without being stereotypically dismissed as being "difficult" or "angry." She told me the onus is on America.

"I think the better question is what does *America* need to know about the biases in healthcare and the treatment of African Americans," Mason-Cooley said. "There is NO WAY Black women, as well as their children, should be dying four to five times the rate as white women do during childbirth. I can't tell you the numerous stories I've heard. I experienced this myself as well. I can't fault myself, but I did not push the issue. Our baby died, and I think it could've been prevented. Wednesday night I told the nurses I was having horrible stomach pains. They 'made note of it.' The next morning our daughter was dead. I will *never* let that happen again. They didn't believe me, and I and my child became yet another statistic."

Mason-Cooley said that she doesn't want to undermine any doctor or nurse, and recognizes that medicine is a noble profession. "But I know people with sickle cell that have actually died from a heart attack because the pain was so excruciating," she tells NBC. "No one took it seriously, and they passed away. So it's gotta stop. We're asking you to listen to us."

So until we dismantle systemic racism and the patriarchy, what can women, especially women of color, do to protect themselves at the doctor's office?

Writer and health coach Ragen Chastain spells it out clearly. "It's your body," she wrote in *Medium*. "There may have been a time when it made sense to put healthcare providers completely in charge of our health, but that's no longer the case. We need to be part of our healthcare team."[10]

Nine Ways to Be Your Own Advocate

1. **Be prepared**: "Being well-prepared for your appointment can maximize the time you have with your doctor and other practitioners," Chastain wrote. "Being informed—and having information at the ready—means that you can expedite the

diagnostic process and give them the maximum possible time to practice their healing modality."[11]

2. **Gather your personal and family health history:** "If you are able to procure records from other facilities where you were treated, that's great information for the physician," Kecia Gaither, MD, an ob-gyn in New York City, told *Glamour.* "Also, have a list of your medications, along with dosages and how long you have been taking it."[12]

3. **Research your provider:** "This is someone you are going to spend a lot of your pregnancy with, and you need to trust them," said Crystal Hawkins, RN, a labor and delivery nurse and birth-rights activist in Philadelphia.[13] "Google them, look at past patient reviews, see if they are on social media, and ask your community groups about them."

   Chastain echoed this point, too. "I don't know why it took me so long to start doing this, but after walking out of one too many appointments with fatphobic medical providers, I realized that I could do some work on the front end and avoid a massive waste of my time and energy," she said. "Now I don't make an appointment with a provider without doing my online research and having a phone conversation."[14]

4. **Inform yourself about pregnancy:** Knowing more about what's "normal" and what is a warning sign can

help you better advocate for yourself when something feels wrong. Black parents should research preeclampsia and preterm labor, two conditions that affect more Black women.[15] When you know more, it helps with your confidence to ask more.[16]

5. **Make a paper trail:** "All women should keep surgical records, most recent annual lab results, history of abnormal lab results, and prenatal care and delivery records," says Temeka Zore, MD, a board-certified ob-gyn in San Francisco.[17]

6. **Change doctors if you don't feel safe:** There is no rule that says you must remain in the care of a provider who doesn't make you feel safe. "Medical training and the 'ivory tower' afford [doctors] a lot of unearned power and privilege in the exam room," Dr. Anjana Sharma, an assistant professor of family community medicine at the University of California, San Francisco School of Medicine, told *Greatist*.[18] "Doctors need to own that power differential, learn trauma-informed care practices, and consider the power dynamics that existed even prior to the clinic visit."

7. **Prepare your partner:** Many people hire a doula—a birth worker who can advocate for you in the delivery room. But if you just have your partner with you, make sure he/she is informed, especially about COVID-related restrictions.

8. **Don't be neglectful during the postpartum period:** "With cardiovascular disease, the postpartum period is a very high-risk period," Jennifer Haythe, MD, a cardiologist and codirector of the Women's Heart Center at Columbia University in New York City, told *Glamour*. "Sometimes people forget that."[19]

9. **It takes a village:** "Your health is a team effort, in which you, not the doctor, play the most important role, so communication is key," Joe Alton, MD, fellow of the American College of Obstetricians and Gynecologists, said.[20]

Conclusion

After being separated from my parents for thirteen months by COVID-19 both in the United States and in Bangladesh, in February 2021 I grabbed a narrow window of opportunity to visit them. For a fleeting moment, it seemed as though South Asia had managed to bring COVID under control with impressive vaccination rollouts and steadily declining death rates.

While I was in Dhaka, I got to make a quick trip with my father to his constituency outside the city. I met and spoke with rural women and local female politicians about the biggest challenges women were facing at the moment and their immediate needs on the ground in the face of the ongoing pandemic.

These conversations made me recall the universality of women's health issues. I listened as woman after woman shared stories about being pressured into cesarean sections at "big city hospitals," their concerns being dismissed because they were female, and how the pandemic has only intensified existing hardships.

When I spoke about my upcoming book, they were proud and

excited for me. But one woman asked me how a book on women's health in America would make any difference for Bangladeshi women. Her question gave me pause. Then I answered that if we can't rectify women's health and human rights in America, women in the rest of the world will effectively be "screwed."

I was reminded of how we are all connected. As women, we share unique bonds from childbirth to the loss of a child, to being dismissed and not being believed. The good and the bad connect us. Sisterhood is truly global, and if there has ever been a time for women to tap into our collective power, it is now because the need to revolutionize women's healthcare is urgent.

After initially excluding pregnant women from clinical trials for the COVID vaccine—trials I have strongly been advocating for all along—in the spring of 2021 experts announced that there is no evidence to suggest that the Pfizer and Moderna COVID-19 vaccines pose risk during pregnancy. The peer-reviewed paper, published by *The New England Journal of Medicine*, used self-reported data from more than 35,691 people who were either pregnant or soon planning to be.[1]

The published results were an extension of a study presented by the CDC's Advisory Committee on Immunization Practices in March 2021, which also found no safety concerns during pregnancy.[2]

So after over a year of being unable to give women a straightforward answer about whether the most anticipated vaccine of recent history was safe for them, causing immeasurable stress and anxiety for pregnant women during a global pandemic over their own safety and that of their unborn children, experts concluded that COVID vaccines are extremely effective at protecting pregnant women. The vaccines also likely provide protection for their babies.

While this is great news, it infuriates me that women and their doctors were left unsure for over a year about what the vaccine might do to them. Clearly, excluding women is just the default response in the medical world.

The delay in including pregnant women in vaccine trials shows how we have no issue testing on women in an uncontrolled environment. This is essentially what happened with the COVID vaccine since women were left to decide for themselves whether to take the huge risk of opting for vaccination.

Even more infuriating, more pregnant women died, experienced complications, or delivered stillborn babies during the pandemic than in previous years. This is according to an analysis of forty studies in seventeen countries published in 2021 by *The Lancet*.[3] Yet, it still wasn't enough for the medical profession to prioritize women's health, especially the lives of pregnant women.

Just in case we didn't get the message, women were reminded once again that our health is simply not a priority when the Johnson & Johnson vaccine was paused in the United States after six cases in which US women reported a "rare and severe" type of blood clot.

As I wrote in my op-ed for CNN, worldwide reaction was immediate to the statistic that only *six* out of six *million* people develop blood clots. This is enraging when we consider that one in one thousand women who take hormonal birth control are at risk for developing blood clots as a matter of course.[4]

Blood clots and death in childbirth remain just two of the risks that American women, especially women of color, are simply expected to accept. Is this the price of being female, even in 2021?

"Yes" is not an option. I remain more convinced than ever that it is past time for women to reclaim "hysteria," to change how we think about it, and to rebrand it as the courage to speak out forcefully with one voice.

It is time to use the power of our voices to revolutionize women's healthcare—in America and around the world. The pandemic has exposed the urgent need for racial justice *and* birth justice. Women's lives matter. The lives of women of color matter.

The time to raise our collective voices is now.

Acknowledgments

Before I even begin naming all the incredible people who helped bring this book out into the world, I have to thank the incomparable Sophia A. Nelson for introducing me to my amazing agent, Leticia Gomez. Thank you for believing in me and this book from the start. Thank you to my editors at Tiller Press, Emily Carelton, Natasha Yglesias, and Leah Miller, for seeing my vision and investing in it.

Growing up, I had too many dreams. From wanting to be a Bollywood star to wanting to be a psychiatrist, the list was endless. But my biggest dream was always to write a book, and it wouldn't have happened without the encouragement, faith, support, guidance, and friendship of some truly incredible people.

First and foremost, I have to thank my mother, Tasmima Hossain, who believed so wholeheartedly in everything and anything I ever set out to do that she made me believe in myself. Thank you for reading everything I wrote. You are the reason I exist, and I love you too much.

To Donna Spisso, my high school AP English teacher: Thank you for teaching me the discipline of writing early on, and for editing this manuscript with me. You are, in so many ways, the unofficial coauthor of this book. Thank you for believing in me and teaching me how to make my words make sense. Thank you for putting up with my love of commas.

Melody Moezzi, there would not have been a book from me without you. Your proofreading and feedback, not to mention all your effort trying to find me an agent, came at a time when I was so close to giving up on becoming an author. Thank you for saving me and my big dream!

During the journey of writing this book, I needed the eyes, ears, and brains of my closest friends more than ever. Thank you to my University of Virginia (UVA) life-crew, Shereen Abdel-Nabi, Ryan Armstrong, and Bilal Qureshi, for being my biggest cheerleaders throughout this process. Thank you for holding my hand.

Bilal, thank you for that boozy lunch at Millie's when we essentially knocked out the overview for my proposal. And thank you, Lizette Baghdadi, for reading one too many terrible book proposals from me. Your guidance and feedback from day one were invaluable.

One of the greatest things about where I live in Washington, DC, are the people—especially the moms. Thank you so much to all my "Wine Night" Chevy Chase/District of Columbia (CCDC) mamas, in neon pink and leopard prints, for one too many drunken conversations about "Anushay's book."

Elizabeth "Lizzie" Worden, thank you for shattering my writer's block with your early proofreading of some terrible writing. I owe you. Thank you to Lydia Weiss and Jaime Shafter for watching my kids so I could write without interruption in the middle of a pandemic. Thank you, ladies, for your endless encouragement and enthusiasm for this book. It held me up and kept me going.

Of course, a huge thank you to Christy Turlington Burns for bringing me back into the maternal health advocacy world where I belong. Thank you to Every Mother Counts (EMC) for being such an incredible organization that guides, inspires, and motivates me every day to do everything I can for women's health.

One of the greatest privileges of my life, especially as a girl who grew up in Bangladesh in the 1980s, was my education. Thank you to my father, Anwar Hossain Manju, for having the foresight to invest in girls' education when others did not. Thank you to the American International School Dhaka (AIS/D) in Bangladesh for providing me with an excellent educational foundation.

Thank you to the University of Virginia (UVA) for expanding my mind and allowing my intellectual curiosity to thrive. Thank you to my sister, Maneeza Hossain, for sending me to writer's camp at UVA and encouraging my writing early on. Thank you to the Institute of Development Studies (IDS) at the University of Sussex in the United Kingdom where I completed my master's in gender and development.

Thank you to all the warrior women who shared their stories with me. Thank you for believing in this book and for your bravery.

And thank you to the women of my motherland, Bangladesh. Bangladeshi women and girls are the strongest women I know. I hope I make you proud.

Notes

Introduction

1. Alison Espach, "What It Really Means When You Call a Woman Hysterical," *Vogue*, March 10, 2017, http://www.vogue.com/article/trump-women-hysteria-and-history.

2. Ursula K. Le Guin, *Dancing at the Edge of the World* (United States: Grove Press, 1997).

3. @MonaEltahawy, Twitter, November 29, 2020, 7:18 a.m., http://www.twitter.com/monaeltahawy/status/126632810067 0976000.

4. Barbara Sadick, "Women Die from Heart Attacks More Often than Men. Here's Why—and What Doctors Are Doing about It," April 1, 2019, *Time*, http://www.time.com/5499872/women-heart-disease/.

5. Diana Baptiste and Yvonne Commodore Mensah, "Black Women and Matters of the Heart," *Johns Hopkins Nursing*, February 14, 2019, https://magazine.nursing.jhu.edu/2019/02/black-women-and-matters-of-the-heart/.

6. Avery Ellfeldt, "Heat and Racism Threaten Birth Outcomes for Women of Color," *Scientific American*, June 22, 2020, http://www.scientificamerican.com/article/heat-and-racism -threaten-birth-outcomes-for-women-of-color/.

Chapter 1:
The First Feminist I Ever Knew

1. In Bangladesh, candidates can run for more than two seats.
2. Dilip Ganguly, "Nature a Familiar Demon in Bangladesh," *Los Angeles Times*, August 4, 1996, https://www.latimes.com /archives/la-xpm-1996-08-04-mn-31126-story.html.
3. "International Conference on Population and Development," United Nations Population Fund (UNFPA), September 5, 1994, https://www.unfpa.org/events/international-conference -population-and-development-icpd.
4. Sneha Barot, "Looking Back While Moving Forward: Marking 20 Years Since the International Conference on Population and Development," Guttmacher Institute, September 2, 2014, http://www.guttmacher.org/gpr/2014/09/looking-back -while-moving-forward-marking-20-years-international -conference-population.
5. Ibid.
6. Rounaq Jahan, "Securing Maternal Health through Comprehensive Reproductive Health Services: Lessons from Bangladesh," *American Journal of Public Health* 97, no. 7 (July 9, 2007): 1186–90, https://www.ncbi.nlm.nih.gov/pmc/articles /PMC1913082/.
7. USAID Global Health Bureau, "Bangladesh: Maternal Deaths Decline by 40 Percent in Less Than 10 Years," USAID, March

11, 2011, https://blog.usaid.gov/2011/03/bangladesh-maternal
-deaths-decline-by-40-percent-in-less-than-10-years/.

Chapter 2:
A Bangladeshi Girl on Capitol Hill

1. "Lifting the Veil: The Shocking Story of How the Taliban Brutalized the Women of Afghanistan. How Much Better Will Their Lives Be Now?," *Time*, December 3, 2001, http://content.time.com/time/covers/0,16641,20011203,00.html.

2. James Gerstenzang and Lisa Getter, "Laura Bush Addresses State of Afghan Women," *Los Angeles Times*, November 18, 2001, http://www.latimes.com/archives/la-xpm-2001-nov-18 -mn-5602-story.html.

3. Michael Bearden, "Afghanistan, Graveyard of Empires," *Foreign Affairs*, November/December 2001, http://www .foreignaffairs.com/articles/afghanistan/2001-11-01/afghani stan-graveyard-empires.

4. Hannah Ritchie, "How Many Women Die in Childbirth?," Our World in Data, September 16, 2019, http://www.our worldindata.org/how-many-women-die-in-childbirth.

5. "The U.S. Government and International Family Planning & Reproductive Health Efforts," Global Health Policy, Kaiser Family Foundation (KFF), July 30, 2019, http://www.kff.org /global-health-policy/fact-sheet/the-u-s-government-and -international-family-planning-reproductive-health-efforts/.

6. Marian L. Lawson and Emily M. Morgenstern, "Foreign Assistance: An Introduction to US Programs and Policy," Congressional Research Service (CRS), April 30, 2020, http:// crsreports.congress.gov/product/pdf/R/R40213.

7. Zara Ahmed, "The Unprecedented Expansion of the Global Gag Rule: Trampling Rights, Health and Free Speech," Guttmacher Institute, April 28, 2020, http://www.guttmacher .org/gpr/2020/04/unprecedented-expansion-global-gag -rule-trampling-rights-health-and-free-speech.

8. Ibid.

9. Rebecca Grant, "Trump's Massive Expansion of the Global Gag Rule Will Kill Women, Advocates Warn," *Vice*, January 25, 2017, http://www.vice.com/en/article/ywmddk/trumps -massive-expansion-of-the-global-gag-rule-will-kill-women -advocates-warn.

10. "Abortions in Africa Increased During 'Global Gag Rule,' Stanford University Study Shows," Kaiser Family Foundation (KFF), September 30, 2011, http://www.kff.org/news -summary/abortions-in-africa-increased-during-global-gag -rule-stanford-university-study-shows/.

11. Ibid.

12. Ibid.

13. "MSF Welcomes Reversal of the Global Gag Rule on Safe Abortion," Médecins Sans Frontières (MSF), January 29, 2021, https://www.msf.org/us-must-step-safe-abortion-efforts -and-access.

14. Ibid.

15. Elizabeth Noble, "New Estimates Show Worldwide Decrease in Unintended Pregnancies," news release, Guttmacher Institute, July 23, 2020, http://www.guttmacher.org/news -release/2020/new-estimates-show-worldwide-decrease -unintended-pregnancies.

16. "Just the Numbers: The Impact of U.S. International Family Planning Assistance, 2016," Guttmacher Institute, May 25,

2016, http://www.guttmacher.org/article/2016/05/just-numbers
-impact-us-international-family-planning-assistance.

17. Serra Sippel, "The Collateral Damage of Trump's Global Gag
Rule: LGBT Rights," *Advocate*, June 5, 2018, http://www
.advocate.com/commentary/2018/6/05/collateral-damage
-trumps-global-gag-rule-lgbt-rights.

18. Barbara Crossette, "United Nations Population Fund Thriving
as It Praises an American Who Kept U.S. Interest Alive," *Ms.*,
October 6, 2020, http://www.msmagazine.com/2020/10/06
/united-nations-population-fund-thriving-as-it-praises-an
-american-who-kept-u-s-interest-alive/.

19. Ibid.

Chapter 3:
A Tale as Old as Time

1. Jaclyn Friedman, "Deadly Silence: What Happens When
We Don't Believe Women," *Guardian*, January 21, 2020,
http://www.theguardian.com/lifeandstyle/2020/jan/21/what
-happens-when-we-dont-believe-women.

2. Camille Noe Pagán, "When Doctors Downplay Women's
Health Concerns," *New York Times*, May 3, 2018, http://www
.nytimes.com/2018/05/03/well/live/when-doctors-down
play-womens-health-concerns.html.

3. Ashley Boynes Shuck, "Is There a Gender Bias Against Female Patients?" *Healthline*, March 30, 2017, http://www
.healthline.com/health-news/gender-bias-against-female
-pain-patients.

4. Consumer Reports, "Is Bias Keeping Female, Minority Patients from Getting Proper Care for Their Pain?" *Washington
Post*, July 29, 2019, http://www.washingtonpost.com/health

/is-bias-keeping-female-minority-patients-from-getting
-proper-care-for-their-pain/2019/07/26/9d1b3a78-a810-
11e9-9214-246e594de5d5_story.html.

5. Ibid.

6. Ibid.

7. Maria Aspan, "'We Can't Ever Go to the Doctor with Our
Guard Down: Why Black Women Are 40% More Likely to
Die of Breast Cancer," *Fortune*, June 30, 2020, http://www
.fortune.com/2020/06/30/black-women-breast-cancer
-mortality-racism-healthcare-pandemic.

8. "Maternal Mortality: An American Crisis," CBS News,
August 5, 2018, http://www.cbsnews.com/news/maternal
-mortality-an-american-crisis/.

9. Asia Keyes, in-person interview with the author, June 15, 2020.

10. Vidya Rao, "'You Are Not Listening to Me': Black Women
on Pain and Implicit Bias in Medicine," *Today*, July 27, 2020,
http://www.today.com/health/implicit-bias-medicine-how
-it-hurts-black-women-t187866.

12. Amy Mason-Cooley, email correspondence with the author,
December 30, 2020.

13. John Eligon, "Black Doctor Dies of Covid-19 After Complaining of Racist Treatment," *New York Times*, December 23,
2020, http://www.nytimes.com/2020/12/23/us/susan-moore
-black-doctor-indiana.html.

14. "'This Is How Black People Get Killed.' Dr. Susan Moore
Dies of COVID After Decrying Racist Care," *Democracy Now!*, December 30, 2020, http://www.youtube.com
/watch?v=7v1Oyp_bBGk.

15. Fenit Nirappil, "A Black Doctor Alleged Racist Treatment
Before Dying of Covid-19: 'This Is How Black People Get

Killed,'" *Washington Post*, December 24, 2020, http://www
.washingtonpost.com/health/2020/12/24/covid-susan-moore
-medical-racism.

16. Ibid.

17. Ibid.

18. Jessica Firger, "Why Do Doctors Ignore Signs of Heart At-
    tacks in Women?" *New York Post*, February 26, 2018, https://
    www.nypost.com/2018/02/26/why-do-doctors-ignore-signs
    -of-heart-attacks-in-women/.

19. Ibid.

20. ABC News, "Woman Who Suffered 3 Heart Attacks at Age
    40 Wants Women to Know This About Heart Disease," *Good
    Morning America*, February 2, 2018, http://www.goodmorning
    america.com/wellness/story/woman-suffered-heart-attacks
    -age-40-women-heart-52740707.

21. "American Heart Association Wants Women To 'Go Red' on
    Friday," *CBS Miami*, February 2, 2018, https://miami.cbslocal
    .com/2018/02/02/american-heart-association-go-red/.

22. Tressie McMillan Cottom, "I Was Pregnant and in Cri-
    sis. All the Doctors and Nurses Saw Was an Incompetent
    Black Woman," *Time*, January 8, 2019, http://www.time
    .com/5494404/tressie-mcmillan-cottom-thick-pregnancy
    -competent/.

23. Ibid.

24. Ibid.

25. Ibid.

26. Ibid.

27. Ibid.

28. Delan Devakumar, Sujitha Selvarajah, and Geordan Shan-
    non, "Racism, the Public Health Crisis We Can No Longer

Ignore, *The Lancet*, June 11, 2020, https://www.thelancet.com /journals/lancet/article/PIIS0140-6736(20)31371-4/fulltext.

29. Zinzi D. Bailey, Justin M. Feldman, and Mary T. Bassett, "How Structural Racism Works—Racist Policies as a Root Cause of U.S. Racial Health Inequities," *The New England Journal of Medicine*, December 16, 2020, http://www.nejm .org/doi/full/10.1056/NEJMms2025396.

30. Dr. Tina Sacks, email correspondence with the author, December 8, 2020.

31. Nina Martin and Renee Montagne, "Black Mothers Keep Dying After Giving Birth. Shalon Irving's Story Explains Why," *All Things Considered*, National Public Radio (NPR), December 7, 2017, http://www.npr.org /2017/12/07/568948782/black-mothers-keep-dying-after -giving-birth-shalon-irvings-story-explains-why.

32. "Racial and Ethnic Disparities Continue in Pregnancy-Related Deaths," press release, Centers for Disease Control and Prevention (CDC), September 5, 2019, http:/www.cdc .gov/media/releases/2019/p0905-racial-ethnic-disparities -pregnancy-deaths.html.

33. Dr. Tina Sacks, email, December 8, 2020.

Chapter 4:
Invisible Conditions

1. Shereen Abdel-Nabi, interview with the author, January 18, 2021.

2. Margaret Jaworski, "My Story: Padma Lakshmi Talks To *PPM* about Living with the Emotional and Physical Toll of Endometriosis," *Practical Pain Management* (*PPM*), October

18, 2018, http://www.practicalpainmanagement.com/patient
/conditions/pelvic-pain/story-padma-lakshmi-talks-ppm
-about-living-emotional-physical-toll.

3. Ibid.

4. Ibid.

5. Ibid.

6. Ibid.

7. Ibid.

8. Ibid.

9. Alicia Lopez, in-person interview with the author, October
16, 2019.

10. Ibid.

11. Catherine Rakowski, email interview with the author, January
8, 2021.

12. Ibid.

13. Ibid.

14. Amal Abdel-Rahman, in-person interview with the author,
November 6, 2019.

15. Ibid.

16. Maya Dusenbery, *Doing Harm: The Truth about How Bad
Medicine and Lazy Science Leave Women Dismissed, Misdiagnosed, and Sick* (New York: HarperOne, 2018).

17. "How 'Bad Medicine' Dismisses and Misdiagnoses Women's
Symptoms," interview by Terry Gross, *Fresh Air*, National
Public Radio (NPR), March 27, 2018, https://www.npr.org
/transcripts/597159133.

18. Ibid.

19. Ryan Prior, "Women Face Struggles As Patients With Covid-
19—And Beyond," CNN, October 23, 2020, https://www

.cnn.com/2020/10/23/health/womens-health-maya-dusenbery
-wellness/index.html.

20. Druv Khullar, "Even as the U.S. Grows More Diverse, the
Medical Profession Is Slow to Follow," *Washington Post*, September 23, 2018, http://www.washingtonpost.com/national
/health-science/even-as-the-us-grows-more-diverse-the
-medical-profession-is-slow-to-follow/2018/09/21/6e048d66
-aba4-11e8-a8d7-0f63ab8b1370_story.html.

21. Fariss Samarrai, "Study Links Disparities in Pain Management to Racial Bias," *UVA Today*, April 4, 2016, http://news
.virginia.edu/content/study-links-disparities-pain-manage
ment-racial-bias.

22. Gabrielle Jackson, "Why Don't Doctors Trust Women? Because They Don't Know Much About Us," *Guardian*, September 1, 2019, http://www.theguardian.com/books/2019
/sep/02/why-dont-doctors-trust-women-because-they-dont
-know-much-about-us.

23. Ibid.

24. Ibid.

25. Ibid.

26. Cecilia Tasca, Mariangela Rapetti, Mauro Giovanni Carta,
and Bianca Fadda, "Women and Hysteria in the History of
Mental Health," National Center for Biotechnology Information (NCBI), October 19, 2012, http://www.ncbi.nlm.nih
.gov/pmc/articles/PMC3480686/.

27. Ibid.

28. Ibid.

29. Maria Cohut, "The Controversy of 'Female Hysteria,'" *Medical News Today*, October 13, 2020, http://www.medicalnews
today.com/articles/the-controversy-of-female-hysteria.

30. Gabrielle Jackson, "Female Problem: How Male Bias in Medical Trials Ruined Women's Health," *Guardian*, November 13, 2019, http://www.theguardian.com/lifeandstyle/2019/nov/13/the-female-problem-male-bias-in-medical-trials.

31. Ibid.

32. "How 'Bad Medicine' Dismisses and Misdiagnoses."

Chapter 5:
We Don't Know What We Don't Know

1. Dusenbery, *Doing Harm*.

2. Gabrielle Jackson, email correspondence with the author, December 22, 2020.

3. Melody Moezzi, email correspondence with the author, November 24, 2020.

4. Carolyn M. Mazure and Daniel P. Jones, "Twenty Years and Still Counting: Including Women as Participants and Studying Sex and Gender in Biomedical Research," National Center for Biotechnology Information (NCBI), October 26, 2015, http://www.ncbi.nlm.nih.gov/pmc/articles/PMC4624369/.

5. Katherine A. Liu and Natalie A. Dipietro Mager, "Women's Involvement in Clinical Trials: Historical Perspective and Future Implications," National Center for Biotechnology Information (NCBI), March 15, 2016, http://www.ncbi.nlm.nih.gov/pmc/articles/PMC4800017/.

6. Roni Caryn Rabin, "Health Researchers Will Get $10.1 Million to Counter Gender Bias in Studies," *New York Times*, September 23, 2014, http://www.nytimes.com/2014/09/23/health/23gender.html.

7. Jackson, "Female Problem."

8. "Making Women's Health Mainstream: A History," Society for Women's Health Research, accessed May 2, 2021, http://www.swhr.org/about/history/timeline/.

9. Jackson, "Female Problem."

10. "Doctors Confirm Benefits of Aspirin," *New York Times*, July 20, 1989, https://www.nytimes.com/1989/07/20/us/health-doctors-confirm-benefits-of-aspirin.html.

11. Trisha Flynn, "Female Trouble," *Chicago Tribune*, October 29, 1986, https://www.chicagotribune.com/news/ct-xpm-1986-10-29-8603210488-story.html.

12. Mazure and Jones, "Twenty Years and Still Counting."

13. Ibid.

14. Suk Kyeong Lee, "Sex as an Important Biological Variable in Biomedical Research," National Center for Biotechnology Information (NCBI), April 30, 2018, http://www.ncbi.nlm.nih.gov/pmc/articles/PMC5933211/.

15. Rabin, "Health Researchers."

16. Karlyn Q., "What Is the 'Gender Pain Gap'?" Scientista, July 2, 2019, http://www.scientistafoundation.com/career-blog/what-is-the-gender-pain-gap.

17. Brian Resnick, "Genetics Has Learned a Ton—Mostly About White People. That's a Problem," *Vox*, October 27, 2018, http://www.vox.com/science-and-health/2018/10/22/17983568/dna-tests-precision-medicine-genetics-gwas-diversity-all-of-us.

18. Jane L. Delgado and Edward Abrahams, "Diversity in Clinical Trials Defines Good Science and Better Medicine," *Stat*, January 17, 2019, http://www.statnews.com/2019/01/17/diversity-clinical-trials-good-science-better-medicine/.

19. Aspan, "'We Can't Ever Go to the Doctor with Our Guard Down.'"

20. Kai Falkenberg, "FDA Takes Action on Ambien; Concedes Women at Greater Risk," *Forbes*, January 10, 2013, https://www.forbes.com/sites/kaifalkenberg/2013/01/10/fda-takes-action-on-ambien-concedes-women-at-greater-risk/.

21. Elizabeth Cooney, "Females Still Routinely Left Out of Biomedical Research—And Ignored in Analyses of Data," *Stat*, June 9, 2020, http://www.statnews.com/2020/06/09/females-are-still-routinely-left-out-of-biomedical-research-and-ignored-in-analyses-of-data/.

22. Ibid.

23. "Gender Matters: Heart Disease Risk in Women," Harvard Health Publishing, March 25, 2017, www.health.harvard.edu/heart-health/gender-matters-heart-disease-risk-in-women.

24. Ibid.

25. "Heart Disease in African American Women," American Heart Association, February 1, 2021, http://www.goredfo rwomen.org/en/about-heart-disease-in-women/facts/heart-disease-in-african-american-women.

26. William A. Haseltine, "19% of People Infected with COVID in the US Are Healthcare Professionals. Almost Three Quarters of Them Are Women," *Forbes*, April 15, 2020, https://www.forbes.com/sites/williamhaseltine/2020/04/15/19-of-people-infected-with-covid-in-the-us-are-healthcare-professionals-almost-three-quarters-of-them-are-women/.

27. Laura D. Zambrano et. al, "Update: Characteristics of Symptomatic Women of Reproductive Age with Laboratory-Confirmed SARS-CoV-2 Infection by Pregnancy Status—United States, January 22–October 3, 2020," Centers for Disease Control and Prevention (CDC), November 6, 2020, http://www.cdc.gov/mmwr/volumes/69/wr/mm6944e3.htm.

28. Zambrano et al., "Characteristics of Symptomatic Women."

29. William A. Haseltine, "Pregnant Women Are at Higher Risk for Severe Covid-19 and Death," *Forbes*, November 9, 2020, https://www.forbes.com/sites/williamhaseltine/2020/11/09/pregnant-women-are-at-higher-risk-for-severe-covid-19-and-death/.

30. Laurel Wamsley, "Pregnant People Haven't Been Part of Vaccine Trials. Should They Get the Vaccine?" National Public Radio (NPR), December 11, 2020, https://www.npr.org/2020/12/11/945196602/pregnant-people-havent-been-part-of-vaccine-trials-should-they-get-the-vaccine.

31. Ibid.

32. Alison Bowen, "Should Pregnant Women Get a COVID-19 Vaccine? What About Women Considering Pregnancy? Guidance Is Hard to Find Because Trials Exclude Pregnancy," *Chicago Tribune*, December 2, 2020, http://www.chicagotribune.com/coronavirus/ct-life-covid-pregnant-women-becoming-pregnant-vaccine-tt-20201202-xl4jvwjoqvfhfpciigjetcef5a-story.html.

33. American College of Obstetricians and Gynecologists (ACOG), "Maternal Immunization Task Force and Partners Urge that COVID-19 Vaccine Be Available to Pregnant Individuals," February 3, 2021, https://www.acog.org/news/news-releases/2021/02/maternal-immunization-task-force-and-partners-urge-that-covid-19-vaccine-be-available-to-pregnant-individuals.

34. William Wan, "Pregnant Women Are More Likely to Die from the Coronavirus, Though Risk Remains Small," *Washington Post*, November 2, 2020, http://www.washingtonpost.com/health/2020/11/02/covid-pregnant-women-death/.

35. Miriam Berger, "Medical Research Again Leaves Pregnant Women Waiting for a Vaccine—This Time for Coronavirus," *Washington Post*, December 10, 2020, http://www.washingtonpost.com/world/2020/12/10/pregnant-women-are-excluded-initial-covid-19-vaccinations-highlighting-worldwide-research-gap/.

36. Holly Honderich, "Will Pregnant Women Receive the Covid-19 Vaccine? It Depends," British Broadcasting Corporation (BBC), December 22, 2020, http://www.bbc.com/news/world-us-canada-55340244.

37. Wamsley, "Pregnant People Haven't Been Part of Vaccine Trials.

38. Berger, "Medical Research Again Leaves Pregnant Women."

39. Miriam Fauzia, "Fact Check: Pregnant Women Do Receive Vaccines, but More Study Needed on COVID-19 Shot," *USA Today*, December 29, 2020, http://www.usatoday.com/story/news/factcheck/2020/12/29/fact-check-pregnant-women-get-vaccines-study-needed-covid-19-shot/3992718001/.

40. Aubrey Whelan, "The COVID-19 Vaccine Wasn't Tested in Pregnancy, but Experts Say It's Still Worth Considering if You're Expecting," *Philadelphia Inquirer*, December 14, 2020, http://www.inquirer.com/health/coronavirus/pregnancy-covid-vaccine-healthcare-workers-20201214.html.

41. Megan Henry and Karen Weintraub, "For Pregnant and Nursing Women, Risks of COVID-19 Probably Outweigh Risk of Vaccine, Experts Say," *Columbus Dispatch*, December 23, 2020, https://www.dispatch.com/story/news/coronavirus/2020/12/23/pregnant-nursing-women-risks-covid-19-coronavirus-outweigh-risk-vaccine-experts-say/3955907001.

42. Ibid.

43. Ibid.

44. Maria Navarro, phone interview with the author, October 25, 2020.

45. Ebony Marcelle, email correspondence with the author, January 14, 2021.

46. "Gayle Jordan," phone interview with the author, October 25, 2020.

47. Glenda Ruiz, phone interview with the author, November 10, 2020.

48. Melissa Lu, phone interview with the author, November 8, 2020.

49. Sandee LaMotte, "Pregnant Women Should Get Covid-19 Vaccine, US Doctors Say, Despite Conflicting International Advice," CNN, January 30, 2021, http://www.cnn.com/2021/01/29/health/pregnancy-covid-vaccine-wellness/index.html.

50. Ibid.

51. Sarah Toy, "WHO Recommends Against Moderna, Pfizer Vaccines for Most Pregnant Women," *Wall Street Journal*, January 27, 2021, http://www.wsj.com/articles/who-recommends-against-moderna-pfizer-vaccines-for-most-pregnant-women-11611775138.

52. Ibid.

53. Katharine Gammon, "A Pandemic Pregnancy Is a More Dangerous Pregnancy," *The Atlantic*, December 24, 2020, http://www.theatlantic.com/health/archive/2020/12/covid-19-pregnancy/617507/.

54. Ibid.

55. Frances Stead Sellers, "Pregnant Women Agonize Over Whether to Get Coronavirus Vaccine," *Washington Post*, January 1, 2021, http://www.washingtonpost.com/health/pregnant

-women-covid-vaccine/2021/01/01/b62ff88a-4492-11eb
-b0e4-0f182923a025_story.html.

56. Melanie Taylor et al., "Inclusion of Pregnant Women in COVID-19 Treatment Trials: A Review and Global Call to Action," *The Lancet*, December 16, 2020, https://www.thelancet .com/journals/langlo/article/PIIS2214-109X(20)30484-8 /fulltext.

57. Sellers, "Pregnant Women Agonize."

58. Helen Lewis, "The Coronavirus Is a Disaster for Feminism," *The Atlantic*, March 19, 2020, http://www.theatlantic.com /international/archive/2020/03/feminism-womens-rights -coronavirus-covid19/608302/.

59. Ibid.

60. Ibid.

61. Ibid.

62. Julie Kashen, "How COVID-19 Sent Women's Workforce Progress Backward," Center for American Progress, October 30, 2020, http://www.americanprogress.org/issues/women/reports /2020/10/30/492582/covid-19-sent-womens-workforce -progress-backward/.

63. Ibid.

64. Annalyn Kurtz, "The US Economy Lost 140,000 Jobs in December. All of Them Were Held by Women," CNN, January 8, 2021, https://www.cnn.com/2021/01/08/economy/women -job-losses-pandemic/index.html.

65. Hanna Rosin, "The End of the End of Men," *New York*, February 1, 2021, http://www.thecut.com/2021/02/hanna-rosin -end-of-the-end-of-men.html.

66. Ibid.

67. Ibid.

68. Ibid.

69. Ibid.

70. Ibid.

71. Ibid.

72. Ernie Tedeschi, "The Mystery of How Many Mothers Have Left Work Because of School Closings," *New York Times*, October 29, 2020, https://www.nytimes.com/2020/10/29/upshot /mothers-leaving-jobs-pandemic.html.

73. Misty L. Heggeness and Jason M. Fields, "Working Moms Bear Brunt of Home Schooling While Working During COVID-19," United States Census Bureau, August 18, 2020, https://www.census.gov/library/stories/2020/08/parents -juggle-work-and-child-care-during-pandemic.html.

74. Jenesse Miller, "COVID-19 Pandemic Has Hit Women Hard, Especially Working Mothers," USC Dornsife, June 18, 2020, https://dornsife.usc.edu/news/stories/3234/covid-19-pandemic -has-hit-women-hard-especially-working-mothers/.

75. @RachelPatzerPhd, Twitter, March 16, 2020, 9:35 p.m., http://www.twitter.com/rachelpatzerphd/status/1239726900 446191617?lang=en.

76. Margie Davenport et al., "Moms Are Not OK: COVID-19 and Maternal Mental Health," *Frontiers in Global Women's Health*, June 19, 2020, http://www.frontiersin.org/articles /10.3389/fgwh.2020.00001/full.

77. Katharine Gammon, "The Psychic Toll of a Pandemic Pregnancy," *New York Times*, December 16, 2020, http://www .nytimes.com/2020/12/14/parenting/pregnancy/pregnant- with-coronavirus.html.

78. Ibid.

79. Ibid.

80. Ibid.

81. Davenport, "Moms Are Not OK."

82. Ibid.

83. Lynda Hernandez, phone interview with the author, November 24, 2020.

84. Corrine Hudson, phone interview with the author, November 24, 2020.

85. Ibid.

86. Ibid.

87. Ibid.

88. Ibid.

89. Pooja Lakshmin, "Experts Fear Increase in Postpartum Mood and Anxiety Disorders," *New York Times*, May 27, 2020, https://www.nytimes.com/2020/05/27/parenting/coronavirus -postpartum-depression-anxiety.html.

90. Ines Moina, phone interview with the author, November 30, 2020.

91. Nadiya Hussein, phone interview with the author, November 30, 2020.

92. Kimberly Shaffer, phone interview with the author, November 30, 2020.

93. @TanzinaVega, Twitter, 14 January, 2021, http://www.twitter .com/tanzinavega/status/1349846918726361088?lang=en.

94. Ibid.

95. Anne Helen Petersen, "'Other Countries Have Social Safety Nets. The U.S. Has Women,'" *Culture Study*, November 11, 2020, http://annehelen.substack.com/p/other-countries-have -social-safety.

96. Ibid.

97. Ibid.

98. Ibid.

99. Ibid.

100. Claire Cain Miller, "When Schools Closed, Americans Turned to Their Usual Backup Plan: Mothers," *New York Times*, November 17, 2020, http://www.nytimes.com/2020/11/17/upshot/schools-closing-mothers-leaving-jobs.html.

101. Jessica Valenti, "Women Will Bear the Burden of Getting Our Aging Parents Vaccinated," *Medium*, January 15, 2021, http://gen.medium.com/the-job-of-making-sure-our-senior-parents-are-vaccinated-will-fall-on-women-6a95d30ab4d1.

102. Ibid.

103. Sasha Pezenik, "Women More Likely to Experience Depression, Anxiety, New CDC Data Shows," ABC News, September 24, 2020, http://abcnews.go.com/Health/women-experience-depression-anxiety-cdc-data-shows/story?id=73167309.

104. Ibid.

105. Shefali Luthra, "Job Insecurity, Child Care: Moms Reporting Psychological Distress Amid Coronavirus Pandemic," *USA Today*, August 7, 2020, updated August 16, 2020, http://www.usatoday.com/story/news/politics/2020/08/07/coronavirus-pandemic-leads-explosion-depression-anxiety-women-trans/3309916001/.

106. Brandi Jackson and Aderonke B. Pedersen, "Opinion: Facing Both Covid-19 and Racism, Black Women Are Carrying a Particularly Heavy Burden," *Washington Post*, September 4, 2020, https://www.washingtonpost.com/opinions/2020/09/04

/facing-both-covid-19-racism-black-women-are-carrying
-particularly-heavy-burden/.

107. Ibid.

108. Lynya Floyd, "Black Women Are Facing an Overwhelming Mental Health Crisis," *Prevention*, November 6, 2020, http:// www.prevention.com/health/mental-health/a33686468 /black-women-mental-health-crisis/.

109. Ibid.

110. Ibid.

111. Ibid.

112. Sherri Williams, "After 40 Years of Staying Silent about My Depression, Last Week I Told the Whole World," *Self*, May 31, 2017, http://www.self.com/story/talking-about-dealing-with -depression.

113. Ibid.

114. Sherri Williams, "Racism and the Invisible Struggle of Mental Health in the Black Community," *Self*, May 22, 2017, http:// www.self.com/story/racism-mental-health-in-the-black -community?mbid=social_twitter.

115. Ibid.

116. Azza Altiraifi and Nicole Rapfogel, "Mental Health Care Was Severely Inequitable, Then Came the Coronavirus Crisis," Center for American Progress, September 10, 2020, http://www.americanprogress.org/issues/disability/reports /2020/09/10/490221/mental-health-care-severely-inequitable -came-coronavirus-crisis/.

117. Pezenik, "Women More Likely to Experience Depression, Anxiety."

118. Williams, "After 40 Years."

119. Ibid.

120. Pezenik, "Women More Likely to Experience Depression, Anxiety."

121. Zahra Haider, in-person interview with the author, January 11, 2020.

122. Sofia Carratala and Connor Maxwell, "Health Disparities by Race and Ethnicity," Center for American Progress, May 7, 2020, https://www.americanprogress.org/issues/race/reports/2020/05/07/484742/health-disparities-race-ethnicity/.

123. D'Vera Cohn and Jeffrey S. Passel, "A Record 64 Million Americans Live in Multigenerational Households," Pew Research Center, April 5, 2018, http://www.pewresearch.org/fact-tank/2018/04/05/a-record-64-million-americans-live-in-multigenerational-households/.

124. Cohn and Passel, "A Record 64 Million Americans."

125. Alisha Haridasani Gupta, "Why Some Women Call This Recession a 'Shecession,'" New York Times, May 9, 2020, updated May 13, 2020, https://www.nytimes.com/2020/05/09/us/unemployment-coronavirus-women.html.

126. Campbell Robertson and Robert Gebeloff, "How Millions of Women Became the Most Essential Workers in America," New York Times, April 18, 2020, http://www.nytimes.com/2020/04/18/us/coronavirus-women-essential-workers.html.

127. Nina Martin and Bernice Yeung, "'Similar to Times of War': The Staggering Toll of COVID-19 on Filipino Health Care Workers," ProPublica, May 3, 2020, http://www.propublica.org/article/similar-to-times-of-war-the-staggering-toll-of-covid-19-on-filipino-health-care-workers.

128. Ibid.

129. Ibid.

130. Ibid.

131. Luca Powell, "'It's Starting Again': Why Filipino Nurses Dread the Second Wave," *New York Times*, January 15, 2021, http://www.nytimes.com/2021/01/15/nyregion/filipino-nurses-coronavirus.html.

132. Ibid.

133. Ibid.

134. Ibid.

135. Ibid.

136. "Sins of Omission," National Nurses United, accessed January 31, 2021, https://www.nationalnursesunited.org/sites/default/files/nnu/graphics/documents/0920_Covid19_SinsOf Omission_Data_Report.pdf.

137. Ibid.

138. Catherine Powell, "Color of Covid: The Racial Justice Paradox of Our New Stay-at-Home Economy," CNN, April 18, 2020, http://www.cnn.com/2020/04/10/opinions/covid-19-people-of-color-labor-market-disparities-powell/index.html.

139. Ibid.

140. Ibid.

141. Ibid.

142. Ibid.

143. Laura D. Lindberg, Alicia VandeVusse, Jennifer Mueller, and Marielle Kirstein, "Early Impacts of the COVID-19 Pandemic: Findings from the 2020 Guttmacher Survey of Reproductive Health Experiences," Guttmacher Institute, June 2020, http://www.guttmacher.org/report/early-impacts-covid-19-pandemic-findings-2020-guttmacher-survey-reproductive-health.

144. Melissa S. Kearney and Phillip Levine, "Half a Million Fewer Children? The Coming COVID Baby Bust," Brookings, June

15, 2020, http://www.brookings.edu/research/half-a-million
-fewer-children-the-coming-covid-baby-bust/.

145. Eliana Dockterman, "Women Are Deciding Not to Have Babies Because of the Pandemic. That's Bad for All of Us," *Time*,
October 15, 2020, http://www.time.com/5892749/covid-19
-baby-bust/.

146. Lindberg et al., "Early Impacts of the COVID-19 Pandemic."

147. Dockterman, "Women Are Deciding."

148. Kearney and Levine, "Half a Million Fewer Children?"

149. Dockterman, "Women Are Deciding."

150. Lindberg et al., "Early Impacts of the COVID-19 Pandemic."

151. National Statistics, National Coalition Against Domestic
Violence (NCADV), accessed January 27, 2021, https://www
.ncadv.org/STATISTICS.

152. N. Jamiyla Chisholm, "COVID-19 Creates Added Danger
for Women in Homes with Domestic Violence," *Colorlines*,
March 27, 2020, http://www.colorlines.com/articles/covid
-19-creates-added-danger-women-homes-domestic-violence.

153. Robyn Bleiweis and Osub Ahmed, "Ensuring Domestic
Violence Survivors' Safety," Center for American Progress,
August 10, 2020, http://www.americanprogress.org/issues
/women/reports/2020/08/10/489068/ensuring-domestic
-violence-survivors-safety/.

154. Eve Valera, "When Lockdown Is Not Actually Safer: Intimate Partner Violence During COVID-19," Harvard Health
Publishing, July 7, 2020, http://www.health.harvard.edu
/blog/when-lockdown-is-not-actually-safer-intimate-partner
-violence-during-covid-19-2020070720529.

155. Ibid.

156. Laila Qureshi, phone interview with the author, December 11, 2020.

157. Ibid.

158. Ibid

159. Tanisha Leaf, phone interview with the author, December 21, 2020.

160. Brad Boserup, Mark McKenney, and Adel Elkbuli, "Alarming Trends in US Domestic Violence During the COVID-19 Pandemic," *American Journal of Emergency Medicine* 38, no. 12, December 1, 2020, http://www.ajemjournal.com/article /S0735-6757(20)30307-7/fulltext.

161. Boserup, McKenney, and Elkbuli, "Alarming Trends in US Domestic Violence."

162. "Understanding Intimate Partner Violence," Harvard Health Publishing, January 2021, http://www.health.harvard.edu /womens-health/understanding-intimate-partner-violence.

163. Mélissa Godin, "As Cities Around the World Go on Lockdown, Victims of Domestic Violence Look for a Way Out," *Time*, March 18, 2020, http://www.time.com/5803887 /coronavirus-domestic-violence-victims/.

164. Ibid.

165. "Domestic Violence and COVID-19: When It's Dangerous to Be Stuck at Home," CU Denver News, October 25, 2020, http://news.ucdenver.edu/domestic-violence-and-covid-19 -when-its-dangerous-to-be-stuck-at-home/.

166. Ibid.

167. Godin, "As Cities Around the World Go on Lockdown."

168. Ibid.

169. Ibid.

170. Lisa Geller and Lauren Footman, "Guns, Domestic Violence, and COVID-19 Are a Lethal Combination," Morning Consult, October 27, 2020, http://www.morningconsult.com/opinions/guns-domestic-violence-and-covid-19-are-a-lethal-combination/.

171. Ibid.

172. Ibid.

173. Ibid.

174. Katherine Kam, "Why Domestic Violence Calls Are Surging for Asian American Women Amid the Pandemic," Yahoo! Entertainment, October 1, 2020, http://www.yahoo.com/entertainment/why-domestic-violence-calls-suring-100022994.html.

175. Ibid.

176. Ibid.

177. Ibid.

178. Ibid.

179. Ibid.

180. Kavita Mehra, phone interview and email correspondence, February 3, 2021.

181. Ibid.

182. Kam, "Why Domestic Violence Calls Are Surging."

183. Nicholas Turton, "Attacks Against AAPI Community Continue to Rise During Pandemic," press statement, Stop AAPI Hate, August 27, 2020, http://www.asianpacificpolicyandplanningcouncil.org/wp-content/uploads/PRESS_RELEASE_National-Report_August27_2020.pdf.

184. Ibid.

185. Jessica Gingrich, "When Nowhere Feels Safe: COVID-19, Anti-Asian Racism and Domestic Violence," *Hyphen*, Septem-

ber 25, 2020, http://www.hyphenmagazine.com/blog/2020/09
/when-nowhere-feels-safe-covid-19-anti-asian-racism-and
-domestic-violence.

186. Ibid.

187. Ibid.

188. Ibid.

189. "The Shadow Pandemic: Violence Against Women During COVID-19," UN Women, http://www.unwomen.org /en/news/in-focus/in-focus-gender-equality-in-covid-19 -response/violence-against-women-during-covid-19.

190. Raf Casert and Angela Charlton, "Global Push to End Domestic Violence, Worse Amid COVID-19," Associated Press, November 25, 2020, http://www.apnews.com/article/inter national-news-pandemics-violence-coronavirus-pandemic -france-438ab8d652eddd44ce0e3772d9c755c3.

191. Ibid.

192. Ibid.

193. Megan L. Evans, Margo Lindauer, and Maureen E. Farrell, "A Pandemic within a Pandemic—Intimate Partner Violence During Covid-19," *New England Journal of Medicine*, December 10, 2020, http://www.nejm.org/doi/full/10.1056 /NEJMp2024046.

194. Ibid.

195. "The Biden Plan to End Violence Against Women," Biden/ Harris, accessed May 2, 2021, http://www.joebiden.com/vawa/.

196. "Feminists Applaud the 20th Anniversary of the Violence Against Women Act," Feminist Majority, September 12, 2014, http://www.feministmajority.org/press/feminists-applaud -the-20th-anniversary-of-the-violence-against-women-act/.

197. Ibid.

198. Ibid.

199 Ibid.

200. Ibid.

201. @JoeBiden, Twitter, November 25, 2020, 1:09 p.m., http://www.twitter.com/joebiden/status/1331661301509222401?lang=en.

202. Lewis, "The Coronavirus Is a Disaster for Feminism."

203. Ibid.

204. Ibid.

Chapter 6:
Pregnancy in a Pandemic

1. Roosa Tikkanen, Munira Z. Gunja, Molly FitzGerald, and Laurie Zephyrin, "Maternal Mortality and Maternity Care in the United States Compared to 10 Other Developed Countries," Commonwealth Fund, November, 18, 2020, https://www.commonwealthfund.org/publications/issue-briefs/2020/nov/maternal-mortality-maternity-care-us-compared-10-countries.

2. Ibid.

3. Avital Norman Nathman, "Another Nurse Held My Baby's Head into My Vagina to Prevent Him from Being Delivered," *Cosmopolitan*, August 10, 2016, http://www.cosmopolitan.com/lifestyle/news/a62592/caroline-malatesta-brookwood-childbirth-lawsuit/.

4. Ibid.

5. Ibid.

6. Ibid.

7. Alison Young, "Hospitals Know How to Protect Mothers. They Just Aren't Doing It," *USA Today*, July 26, 2018, up-

dated March 23, 2021, http://www.usatoday.com/in-depth
/news/investigations/deadly-deliveries/2018/07/26/maternal
-mortality-rates-preeclampsia-postpartum-hemorrhage-safety
/546889002/.

8. Ibid.

9. Ibid.

10. Dana Bash, Bridget Nolan, Nelli Black, and Patricia DiCarlo,
"Exclusive: Evelyn Yang Reveals She Was Sexually Assaulted
by Her OB-GYN While Pregnant," CNN, January 17,
2020, http://www.cnn.com/2020/01/16/politics/evelyn-yang
-interview-assault/index.html.

11. Ibid.

12. Ibid.

13. Ibid.

14. Ibid.

15. Ibid.

16. Ibid.

17. Ibid.

18. "Maternal Mortality," World Health Organization (WHO),
September 19, 2019, http://www.who.int/news-room/fact
-sheets/detail/maternal-mortality.

19. Esther Breger, "Paid Leave This Week: 25 Percent of New
Moms Return to Work After Just Two Weeks," *New Republic*,
August 21, 2015, http://newrepublic.com/article/122586/paid
-leave-25-percent-new-moms-return-work-after-just-two
-weeks.

20. "Maternal Mortality Drops 40 Percent in Bangladesh," Measure Evaluation, February 13, 2011, http://www.measure
evaluation.org/our-work/family-planning/maternal-deaths
-down-in-bangladesh.

21. Anushay Hossain, "Making Every Mother Count: Christy Turlington Burns Talks Women's Health and Rights," *Forbes*, July 22, 2013, https://www.forbes.com/sites/world views/2013/07/22/making-every-mother-count-christy -turlington-burns-talks-womens-health-rights/.

22. Ibid.

23. https://www.sxsw.com/.

24. Emily Woodruff, "Louisiana's Rate of Dying Mothers Should 'Shock Us All,' Official Says; Industry Seeks Answers," Nola.com, August 21, 2019, http://www.nola.com/news /article_444031bc-c460-11e9-bc2a-5375a9f7fbaf.html.

25. Ibid.

26. Ibid.

27. Ibid.

28. Ibid.

29. Ibid.

30. Malika Bilal, in-person interview with the author, August 21, 2019.

31. Nina Martin and Renee Montagne, "Black Mothers Keep Dying After Giving Birth. Shalon Irving's Story Explains Why," *All Things Considered*, National Public Radio (NPR), December 7, 2017, https://www.npr.org/2017/12/07/568948782/black -mothers-keep-dying-after-giving-birth-shalon-irvings-story -explains-why.

32. Ibid.

33. Linda Villarosa, "Myths about Physical Racial Differences Were Used to Justify Slavery—and Are Still Believed by Doctors Today," *New York Times*, August 14, 2019, http://www .nytimes.com/interactive/2019/08/14/magazine/racial-differ ences-doctors.html.

34. Kate Womersley, "Why Giving Birth Is Safer in Britain Than in the U.S.," ProPublica, August 31, 2017, https://www .propublica.org/article/why-giving-birth-is-safer-in-britain -than-in-the-u-s.

35. "Racial and Ethnic Disparities Continue in Pregnancy-Related Deaths," press release, Centers for Disease Control and Prevention (CDC), September 5, 2019, http://www.cdc .gov/media/releases/2019/p0905-racial-ethnic-disparities -pregnancy-deaths.html.

36. Dr. Rachael Overcash, phone interview and email correspondence with the author, January 21, 2021.

37. Betty Islinger, phone interview with the author, September 11, 2020.

38. Parveen Phillips, phone interview with the author, December 5, 2020.

39. Ava Letterman, phone interview with the author, December 5, 2020.

40. Elizabeth Mollard and Amaya Wittmaack, "Experiences of Women Who Gave Birth in US Hospitals During the COVID-19 Pandemic," SAGE Journals, January 12, 2021, http://journals.sagepub.com/doi/full/10.1177/23743735209 81492.

41. Ibid.

42. "Confronting Racism During the Pandemic: James-Conterelli Charts Her Course," Yale School of Nursing, December 17, 2020, http://nursing.yale.edu/news/confronting-racism-during -pandemic-james-conterelli-charts-her-course.

43. Ibid.

44. Ibid.

45. Ibid.

46. Ibid.

47. Ibid.

48. Ibid.

49. Anna North, "America Is Failing Black Moms During the Pandemic," *Vox*, August 10, 2020, http://www.vox.com/2020/8/10/21336312/covid-19-pregnancy-birth-black-maternal-mortality.

50. Ibid.

51. Monica R. McLemore, "COVID-19 Is No Reason to Abandon Pregnant People," *Scientific American*, March 26, 2020, http://blogs.scientificamerican.com/observations/covid-19-is-no-reason-to-abandon-pregnant-people/.

52. Ibid.

53. Monica R. McLemore, email correspondence with the author, January 26, 2021.

54. Gbenga Ogedegbe, Joseph Ravenell, Samrachana Adhikari et al., "Assessment of Racial/Ethnic Disparities in Hospitalization and Mortality in Patients with COVID-19 in New York City," *JAMA Netw Open*, December 4, 2020, http://www.jamanetwork.com/journals/jamanetworkopen/fullarticle/2773538.

55. Ibid.

56. Alexandra Villareal, "New York Mother Dies After Raising Alarm on Hospital Neglect," *Guardian*, May 2, 2020, http://www.theguardian.com/us-news/2020/may/02/amber-rose-isaac-new-york-childbirth-death.

57. Ibid.

58. Ibid.

59. @Radieux_Rose, Twitter, April 17 2020, 10:22 a.m., https://twitter.com/Radieux_Rose/status/1251153973886676994.

60. Alexandra Villarreal, "New York Mother Dies After Raising Alarm on Hospital Neglect," *The Guardian*, May 2, 2020, http://www.theguardian.com/us-news/2020/may/02/amber-rose-isaac-new-york-childbirth-death.

61. Ibid.

62. Ibid.

63. Alyssa Newcomb, "Pregnant 26-Year-Old's Death Sheds Light on Health Care System that Fails Black Mothers," *Today*, July 15, 2020, http://www.today.com/health/death-sha-asia-washington-sheds-light-racial-disparities-black-mothers-t186898.

64. Ibid.

65. Rose Adams, "Protesters Slam Bed-Stuy Hospital After Black Woman Dies During Childbirth," *Brooklyn Paper*, July 9, 2020, http:/www.brooklynpaper.com/they-killed-her-protesters-slam-bed-stuy-hospital-after-black-woman-dies-during-childbirth/.

66. Emily Bobrow, "She Was Pregnant with Twins During Covid. Why Did Only One Survive?" *New York Times*, August 6, 2020, http://www.nytimes.com/2020/08/06/nyregion/childbirth-Covid-Black-mothers.html.

67. Marcia Frellick, "Black Chief Resident Dies After Childbirth, Highlights Tragic Trend," Medscape, October 28, 2020, http://www.medscape.com/viewarticle/939954.

68. Ibid.

69. Minyvonne Burke, "Death of Black Mother after Birth of First Child Highlights Racial Disparities in Maternal Mortality," NBC News, November 6, 2020, http://www.nbcnews.com/news/us-news/death-black-mother-after-birth-first-child-highlights-racial-disparities-n1246841.

70. Ibid.

71. Ibid.

72. @rachelvreeman, Twitter, October 26, 2020, 10:57 a.m., https://www.twitter.com/rachelvreeman/status/1320741328603537408.

73. Donna M. Owens, "Pregnant Women Are Contracting COVID-19 and Dying," *Essence*, November 17, 2020, http://www.essence.com/health-and-wellness/pregnant-mothers-covid-19-dying/.

74. Ibid.

75. Ibid.

76. Ibid.

77. Dr. Joia Crear-Perry, "Black Mamas Matter," *Ms.*, February 1, 2019, http://www.msmagazine.com/2019/02/01/black-mamas-matter/.

78. Kiara Haughton Peasant, "Arika's Final Goodbye," GoFundMe.com, June 2020, http://www.gofundme.com/f/arika039s-final-goodbye.

79. Ibid.

80. Ibid.

Chapter 7:
Seeking Alternatives

1. Rachel Scheier, "Black Women Turn to Midwives to Avoid COVID and 'Feel Cared For,'" *Orlando Medical News*, September 19, 2020, http://www.orlandomedicalnews.com/article/3870/black-women-turn-to-midwives-to-avoid-covid-and-feel-cared-for.

2. Jasmine Garsd, "With COVID-19 Hitting Hospitals Hard, Home Births Are on the Rise," Marketplace, November 20,

2020, http://www.marketplace.org/2020/11/20/with-covid-19 -hitting-hospitals-hard-home-births-are-on-the-rise/.

3. North, "America Is Failing Black Moms."

4. Ibid.

5. Austin Frakt, "When Black Patients See Non-Black Doctors," Harvard Global Health Institute, September 9, 2019, http:// globalhealth.harvard.edu/when-black-patients-see-non -black-doctors/.

6. Tonya Russell, "Mortality Rate for Black Babies Is Cut Dramatically When Black Doctors Care for Them after Birth, Researchers Say," *Washington Post*, January 13, 2021, http://www .washingtonpost.com/health/black-baby-death-rate-cut-by -black-doctors/2021/01/08/e9f0f850-238a-11eb-952e-0c475 972cfc0_story.html.

7. Sophia Rogers, phone interview with the author, January 25, 2021.

8. Misha Hylton, phone interview with the author, December 18, 2020.

9. Courteney Brown, phone interview with the author, December 18, 2020.

10. Jasmine Garsd, "With COVID-19 Hitting Hospitals Hard, Home Births Are on the Rise." Marketplace, November 20, 2020, http://www.marketplace.org/2020/11/20/with-covid-19-hitting -hospitals-hard-home-births-are-on-the-rise.

11. Ibid.

12. Kimiko de Freytas-Tamura, "Pregnant and Scared of 'Covid Hospitals,' They're Giving Birth at Home," *New York Times*, April 21, 2020, http://www.nytimes.com/2020/04/21/ny region/coronavirus-home-births.html.

13. Ibid.

14. Naftulin, "Some Pregnant People Want to Switch to a Home Birth."

15. Jessica Salter, "Home Births Are on the Rise in the UK—Now I'm Opting for One, Too," *Vogue*, November 22, 2020, http://www.vogue.co.uk/mini-vogue/article/home-birth.

16. Ibid.

17. Ibid.

18. Jie Qiao, "What Are the Risks of COVID-19 Infection in Pregnant Women?" *The Lancet*, February 12, 2020, http://www.thelancet.com/journals/lancet/article/PIIS0140-6736(20)30365-2/fulltext.

19. Ibid.

20. Gloria Lopez, phone interview with the author, January 24, 2021.

21. Jasmine Garsd, "With COVID-19 Hitting Hospitals Hard."

22. Kennedy Austin, "End Racial Disparities in Maternal Health, Call a Midwife," Columbia University's Mailman School of Public Health, February 2, 2020, http://www.publichealth.columbia.edu/public-health-now/news/end-racial-disparities-maternal-health-call-midwife.

23. Ibid.

24. Ibid.

25. Kimberly Seals Allers, "The Black Maternal Mortality Crisis Deserves Radical Solutions," *Refinery29*, September 23, 2020, https://www.refinery29.com/en-us/black-maternal-mortality-solutions.

26. Garsd, "With COVID-19 Hitting Hospitals Hard."

27. Allers, "The Black Maternal Mortality Crisis."

28. Ibid.

29. Jennie Joseph, "Black History Month: Midwifery Matters," *Every Mother Counts* (EMC) blog, February 13, 2013, http://

blog.everymothercounts.org/black-history-month-midwifery
-matters-e40c16602ab5.

30. Ibid.

31. Ibid.

32. Alicia D. Bonaparte, "The Persecution and Prosecution of
    Granny Midwives in South Carolina, 1900–1940," Vander-
    bilt University Institutional Repository, July 30, 2007, http://
    ir.vanderbilt.edu/handle/1803/13563.

33. Ibid.

34. Joseph, "Midwifery Matters."

35. North, "America Is Failing Black Moms."

36. Joseph, "Midwifery Matters."

37. Ibid.

38. "Joint Statement of Practice Relations Between Obstetrician-
    Gynecologists and Certified Nurse-Midwives/Certified Mid-
    wives," American College of Obstetricians and Gynecolo-
    gists (ACOG), June 1, 2018, http://www.acog.org/clinical
    -information/policy-and-position-statements/statements-of
    -policy/2018/joint-statement-of-practice-relations-between
    -ob-gyns-and-cnms.

39. North, "America Is Failing Black Moms."

40. Ibid.

41. Sarah Zhang, "The Surgeon Who Experimented on Slaves," *The
    Atlantic*, April 18, 2018, http://www.theatlantic.com/health
    /archive/2018/04/j-marion-sims/558248/.

42. Ibid.

43. Ibid.

44. Sarah Lynch, "Fact Check: Father of Modern Gynecology
    Performed Experiments on Enslaved Black Women," *USA
    Today*, June 20, 2020, http://www.usatoday.com/story/news

/factcheck/2020/06/19/fact-check-j-marion-sims-did-medical
-experiments-black-female-slaves/3202541001/.

45. Camila Domonoske, "'Father of Gynecology,' Who Experimented on Slaves, No Longer on Pedestal in NYC," National
Public Radio (NPR), April 17, 2018, http://www.npr.org
/sections/thetwo-way/2018/04/17/603163394/-father-of
-gynecology-who-experimented-on-slaves-no-longer-on
-pedestal-in-nyc.

46. Ibid.

47. Ibid.

48. Shankar Vendantam, "Remembering Anarcha, Lucy, and
Betsey: The Mothers of Modern Gynecology," *Hidden Brain*,
National Public Radio (NPR), February 7, 2017, http://
www.npr.org/transcripts/513764158.

49. Ibid.

50. Ibid.

51. Ibid.

52. Ibid.

53. Ibid.

54. Sandhya Somashekhar, "The Disturbing Reason Some African American Patients May Be Undertreated for Pain," *Washington Post*, April 4, 2016, http://www.washingtonpost.com
/news/to-your-health/wp/2016/04/04/do-blacks-feel-less
-pain-than-whites-their-doctors-may-think-so/.

55. Domonoske, "'Father of Gynecology.'"

56. Vendantam, "Remembering Anarcha, Lucy, and Betsey."

57. Hannah Recht and Lauren Weber, "Black Americans Are
Getting Vaccinated at Lower Rates than White Americans,"
NBC News, January 16, 2021, http://www.nbcnews.com

/health/health-news/black-americans-are-getting-vaccinated
-lower-rates-white-americans-n1254433.

58. Tina Sacks, "When Black People Are Wary of Vaccine, It's Important to Listen and Understand Why," CNN, December 18, 2020, http://www.cnn.com/2020/12/17/opinions/african -americans-covid-vaccine-sacks/index.html.

59. Ibid.

60. Ibid.

61. Associated Press, "Vaccine Skepticism Lurks in Town Famous for Syphilis Study," VIOA, February 1, 2021, http://www .voanews.com/covid-19-pandemic/vaccine-skepticism-lurks -town-famous-syphilis-study.

62. Ibid.

63. Ibid.

64. Sacks, "When Black People Are Wary of Vaccine."

65. Dr. Kimberly D. Manning, "More Than Medical Mis-trust," *The Lancet*, November 7, 2020, http://www.thelancet .com/journals/lancet/article/PIIS0140-6736(20)32286-8 /fulltext.

66. Ibid.

67. Ibid.

68. Ibid.

69. Ibid.

70. Ibid.

71. Ibid.

72. Wesley Lowery, "Why Minneapolis Was the Breaking Point," *The Atlantic*, June 10, 2020, http://www.theatlantic.com /politics/archive/2020/06/wesley-lowery-george-floyd -minneapolis-black-lives/612391/.

73. Ibid.

74. Maneesh Arora, "How the Coronavirus Pandemic Helped the Floyd Protests Become the Biggest in U.S. History," *Washington Post*, August 5, 2020, http://www.washingtonpost.com /politics/2020/08/05/how-coronavirus-pandemic-helped -floyd-protests-become-biggest-us-history/.

75. Michelle Martin, "Poll: Majority of Americans Say Racial Discrimination Is a 'Big Problem,'" National Public Radio (NPR), June 21, 2020, http://www.npr.org/2020/06/21/881477657 /poll-majority-of-americans-say-racial-discrimination-is-a -big-problem.

76. Ibid.

77. Ibid.

78. Lowery, "Why Minneapolis Was the Breaking Point."

79. Arora, "How the Coronavirus Pandemic Helped the Floyd Protests."

80. Sophia A. Nelson, "Here's How We Seize the Moment George Floyd's Murder Has Created," *Daily Beast*, June 10, 2020, http://www.thedailybeast.com/heres-how-we-seize-the -moment-george-floyds-murder-has-created.

81. Ibid.

82. Ibid.

83. Ibid.

84. Ibid.

85. Monica McLemore, email interview with the author, January 26, 2021.

86. Ibid.

87. Ibid.

88. Bobrow, "She Was Pregnant with Twins."

89. "How Many Black, Brown, & Indigenous People Have to Die Giving Birth?" *Every Mother Counts*, July 25, 2020, http://www.everymothercounts.org/wp-content/uploads/2020/07/everymother-print-2.pdf.

90. Ibid.

91. Ibid.

92. Ibid.

93. Ibid.

94. Ibid.

95. Ibid.

96. Ibid.

97. Ibid.

98. Ibid.

99. Ibid.

100. Ibid.

101. Ibram X. Kendi, *How to Be an Anti-Racist* (New York: Random House, 2019).

102. Ibid.

103. Ibid.

104. Ibid.

105. Friedman, "Deadly Silence."

106. Ibid.

107. Ibid.

108. Ibid.

109. Ibid.

110. Ibid.

111. Ibid.

112. Ibid.

Chapter 8:
How to Be Your Own Best Health Advocate

1. Reshma Saujani, "COVID Has Decimated Women's Careers—We Need a Marshall Plan for Moms, Now," *The Hill*, December 7, 2020, http://www.thehill.com/blogs/congress-blog/politics/529090-covid-has-decimated-womens-careers-we-need-a-marshall-plan-for.

2. Ibid.

3. Ibid.

4. Reshma Saujani, email correspondence with the author, February 3, 2021.

5. Saujani, "COVID Has Decimated Women's Careers."

6. Ibid.

7. Saujani, email, February 3, 2021.

8. Saujani, "COVID Has Decimated Women's Careers."

9. Ibid.

10. Ibid.

11. Ibid.

12. Holly Corbett, "Why Mothers Should Be Considered Essential Workers—And Get Paid," *Forbes*, January 29, 2021, https://www.forbes.com/sites/hollycorbett/2021/01/29/why-mothers-should-be-considered-essential-workers-and-get-paid/.

13. Norah O'Donnell, "'We Are in a Moment of Rage': Inside the Movement to Win Basic Income for Moms," CBS News, February 5, 2021, http://www.cbsnews.com/news/universal-basic-income-moms/.

14. Miriam Zoila Pérez, "Making Pregnancy Safer for Women of Color," *New York Times*, February 14, 2018, http://www.nytimes.com/2018/02/14/opinion/pregnancy-safer-women-color.html.

15. Ibid.

16. Ibid.

17. Ibid.

18. Ibid.

19. Ibid.

20. Ibid.

21. Ibid.

22. Ibid.

23. "'This Is Not a New Crisis': How 1 Midwife Is Working to Change Maternal Mortality Rates," *Today*, April 11, 2019, https://www.today.com/video/-this-is-not-a-new-crisis-how-jennie-joseph-is-working-to-change-maternal-mortality-rates-1488326723774.

24. Ibid.

25. Jennie Joseph, Zoom interview and email correspondence, January 31, 2021.

26. "Jamila Taylor Joins the Century Foundation as Director of Health Care Reform and Senior Fellow," Century Foundation, July 22, 2019, https://www.tcf.org/content/about-tcf/jamila-taylor-joins-century-foundation-director-health-care-reform-senior-fellow/.

27. Jamila Taylor, Zoom interview and email correspondence, January 28, 2021.

28. The IHI Triple Aim is a framework developed by the Institute for Healthcare Improvement that describes an approach to optimizing health system performance. It is IHI's belief that new designs must be developed to simultaneously pursue three dimensions, which we call the "Triple Aim."

29. Nan Strauss, phone interview and email correspondence, January 27, 2021.

Chapter 9:
The Truth about Treatment
for Women of Color

1. Kelly Glass, "What to Say If You're a Black Woman and Your Doctor Won't Listen," *Today*, July 24, 2020, http://www.today.com/health/what-say-if-you-re-black-woman-your-doctor-won-t187769.

2. Ibid.

3. Maya Dusenbery, email correspondence with the author, February 1, 2021.

4. "How 'Bad Medicine' Misdiagnoses and Dismisses Women's Symptoms."

5. Gabrielle Jackson, email correspondence with the author, December 23, 2020.

6. Michael Daniel, "Study Suggests Medical Errors Now Third Leading Cause of Death in the U.S.," Johns Hopkins Medicine, May 3, 2016, https://www.hopkinsmedicine.org/news/media/releases/study_suggests_medical_errors_now_third_leading_cause_of_death_in_the_us.

7. Amy Mason-Cooley, email correspondence with the author, December 30, 2020.

8. Rao, "'You Are Not Listening to Me.'"

9. Ibid.

10. Ibid.

11. Ragen Chastain, "The Complete Guide to Becoming Your Own Medical Advocate," *Medium*, August 27, 2018, http://www.medium.com/better-humans/the-complete-guide-to-becoming-your-own-medical-advocate-ddc658a10a57.

12. Ibid.

13. Nina Bahadur, "How to Advocate for Yourself as a Pregnant Black Woman," *Glamour*, August 18, 2020, http://www
.glamour.com/story/how-to-advocate-for-yourself-as-a
-pregnant-black-woman.

14. Ibid.

15. Chastain, "Complete Guide."

16. Bahadur, "How to Advocate."

17. Jenn Sinrich, "10 Questions You Should Never Be Afraid to Ask Your Doctor," *TheWarmUp*, December 13, 2016, http://
www.classpass.com/blog/2016/12/13/questions-to-ask-your
-doctor/.

18. Bahadur, "How to Advocate."

19. Lauren Krouse, "10 Ways Women Can Advocate for Themselves at the Doctor's Office," *Greatist*, November 24, 2020,
https://www.greatist.com/discover/how-women-can-advocate
-for-themselves-at-the-doctors.

20. Bahadur, "How to Advocate."

21. Alison Goldman, "So, Your Doctor Isn't Listening to You. Here Are 4 Effective Ways to Respond," *Women's Health*, February 12, 2020, http:// www.womenshealthmag.com/health
/a30706664/doctor-patient-relationship-how-to-talk-to
-your-doctor/.

Conclusion

1. Tom T. Shimabukuro, Shin Y. Kim, Tanya R. Myers, and Pedro L. Moro, "Preliminary Findings of mRNA Covid-19 Vaccine Safety in Pregnant Persons," *The New England Journal of Medicine*, April 21, 2021, https://www.nejm.org/doi/full/10.1056
/NEJMoa2104983.

2. Tom Shimabukuro, "COVID-19 vaccine safety update," CDC, March 1, 2021, https://www.cdc.gov/vaccines/acip /meetings/downloads/slides-2021-02/28-03-01/05-covid -Shimabukuro.pdf.

3. Barbara Chmielewska, Imogen Barratt, Rosemary Townsend, Erkan Kalafat, and Jan van der Meulen, "Effects of the COVID-19 pandemic on maternal and perinatal outcomes: A systematic review and meta-analysis," *The Lancet*, https:// www.thelancet.com/journals/langlo/article/PIIS2214 -109X(21)00079-6/fulltext.

4. Anushay Hossain, "J&J Vaccine Pause Prompts a Needed Discussion of Women's Health," CNN, April 14, 2021, https:// www.cnn.com/2021/04/14/opinions/johnson-vaccine-pause -womens-reproductive-health-hossain/index.html.

Index

About the Author

Anushay Hossain is a writer and a feminist policy analyst focusing on women's health legislation. She is a regular on-air guest at CNN, MSNBC, and PBS, and her writing on politics, gender, and race has been published in *Forbes*, CNN.com, the *Daily Beast*, and Medium. Hossain is also the host of the *Spilling Chai* podcast. *The Pain Gap* is her first book.